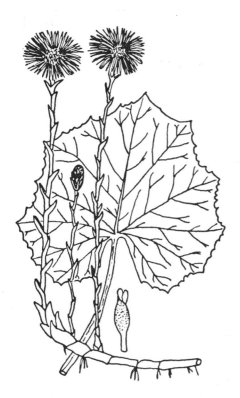

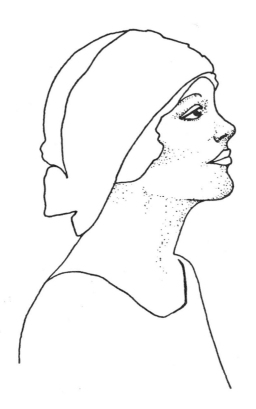

How to make your own HERBAL COSMETICS
The Natural Way to Beauty

LIZ SANDERSON

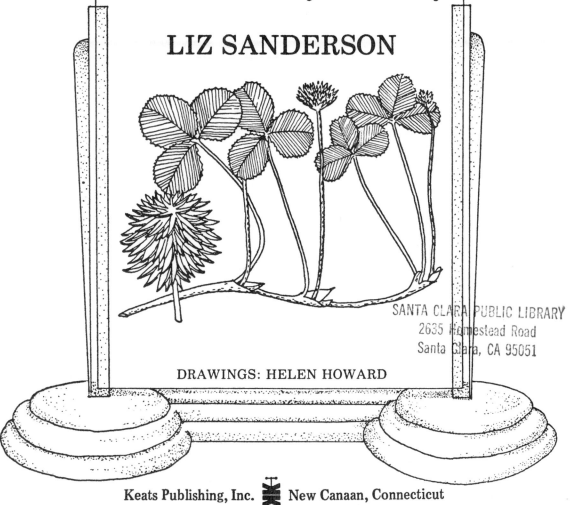

DRAWINGS: HELEN HOWARD

Keats Publishing, Inc. New Canaan, Connecticut

How to Make Your Own Herbal Cosmetics
The Natural Way to Beauty

Published in 1979 by Keats Publishing, Inc.
by arrangement with Latimer New Dimensions Ltd
London, England
Second printing 1993

ISBN: 0-87983-608-3
Library of Congress Catalog Card Number: 78-65301

Printed in the United States of America
Keats Publishing, Inc.
27 Pine Street
Box 876
New Canaan, CT 06840-0876

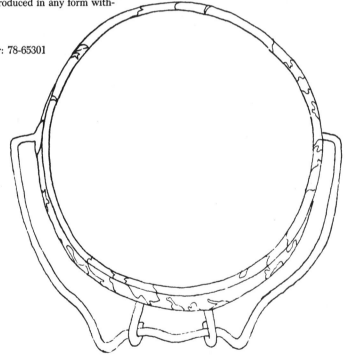

For Hans, who helped me to finish this book
and Snow White who tried to prevent it

CONTENTS

	Introduction	7
1	Where to obtain the ingredients	9
2	Keeping and drying herbs	10
3	How to prepare herbs	12
4	Using herbs in cosmetics	13
5	Face creams	16
6	Skin tonics	19
7	Complexion lotions	21
8	Cleansing methods	23
9	Pimples, spots and acne	26
10	Skin and sun	30
11	Wrinkles	32
12	Mouth, teeth and nose	34
13	Freckles and blotches	37
14	Eyes	39
15	Face masks and compresses	41
16	Body packs	43
17	Beauty baths	44
18	Hair lotions	47
19	Hair rinses	50
20	Hair colourants	52
21	Tips to improve hair condition	57
22	Hands	61
23	Legs and feet	64
24	Perfumes	69
25	Slimming	74
26	Alphabetical herb list	76
27	Glossary of oils, fats, and other unfamiliar substances	102
28	Herbal suppliers	103
29	Bibliography	104
	Index	105

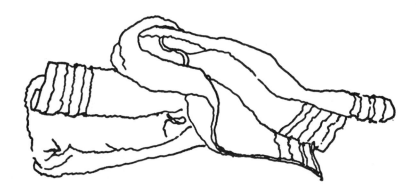

NOTE ON MEASUREMENT

Weights in this book are given in metric units:
measurement of herbs often involves such small
amounts that this is the most precise method.
For those in difficulty, 15 g. = ½ oz., 30 g. =
1 oz., and so on. There is an additional note on
measurement on page 17.

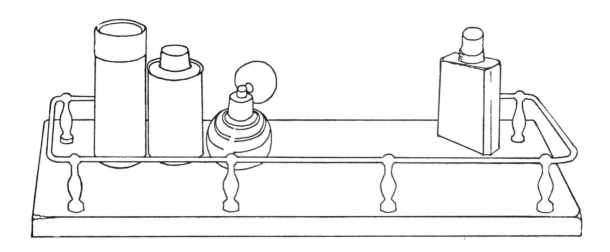

INTRODUCTION

Half a century ago American archaeologists excavated the tomb of Helep Heres I, the mother of the pyramid-builder Cheops. Among the treasures which had been placed in her grave they found a beauty case full of cosmetics. It would seem that beauty has always needed a helping hand. But what is quite new is the amount of money being made by commercial cosmetic firms who frequently package simple substances in exotic pots, bottles and boxes, and who, with the help of advertising, have built up a huge and very lucrative industry.

Unfortunately, some of the chemicals used in commercial products can have the opposite effect to that which was intended. Allergic reactions can be caused by certain perfumes contained in 'beauty' preparations, by irritants in hair dyes and by detergents contained in some cleansing creams. Even more distasteful is the use of hormones, sometimes extracted from placenta and not completely free of health risks. Another undesirable aspect of some commercial cosmetics has been pointed out by anti-vivisectionists and organisations such as 'Beauty without Cruelty': the development of some beauty preparations has involved considerable experimentation on live animals.

The exaggerated claims used to sell these products will, no doubt, give hope to every Cinderella. But let's face it: no anti-wrinkle cream will give you back your youth and no bust lotion will turn a Twiggy into a Jayne Mansfield. The contents of those thick glass bottles and false-bottomed pots can only help to make the best of what is already there.

Natural cosmetics cannot work any miracles either, but they do provide an alternative way to care for your appearance without the disadvantages of commercial preparations. Moreover they can be made at home with very little trouble and considerable savings in costs.

During the last few years the use of herbs in the kitchen and in the sick-room has regained its earlier popularity. In this book I hope to show that herbs are just as much at home in your beauty case. It provides information and recipes to improve the condition of your skin, hair, hands, and so on. Some of the recipes are quite complicated, needing many ingredients and a certain amount of time and effort; others are as simple as making a cup of tea or picking a flower.

7

Obviously, not all the tips and recipes will be suitable for everyone. In any do-it-yourself beauty treatment there is an element of trial and error. But any errors will not have serious consequences when you use natural ingredients and a modicum of common sense. All the recipes in this book have a clearly specified purpose and are worth trying. Here and there you will find old recipes which I have included mainly as curiosities, although occasionally it is suggested that even one of these may be worth a try.

I do hope that men as well as women will use this book. They are certainly no less concerned about their appearance, and both sexes will benefit equally from these often very old and well-tried remedies, and, perhaps most important, will enjoy making and mixing their own herbal cosmetics.

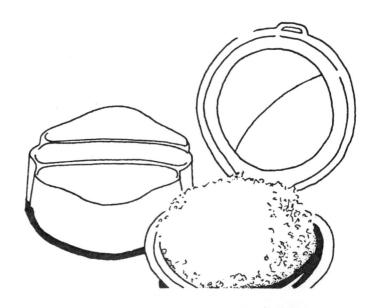

1 WHERE TO OBTAIN THE INGREDIENTS

The various fats and oils, such as spermaceti and sweet almond oil, can be bought at most drugstores. If you go when they are not busy many druggists will weigh small and exact amounts for you. The herbal infusions of witch hazel and rosewater are also available at drugstores. Dried herbs, herbal oils, mixtures and concentrates can often be bought from health food shops and homoeopathic drugstores but the specialist herbal supplier will stock the widest range of products. A list of such specialists will be found on page 103.

Many of the herbs and plants can, of course, be grown easily in the garden or window box, for example, sage, rosemary, lavender, fennel, garlic, cornflowers etc. Others like celandine, speedwell, elder and hawthorn, grow in abundance in the countryside. Even in towns and cities plants like dandelions and nettles can be found on patches of waste ground or open space.

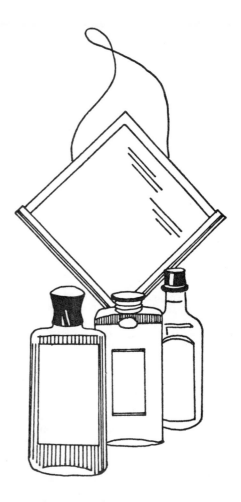

2 KEEPING AND DRYING HERBS

The ideal herb is, of course, young and freshly picked. Even the most carefully dried herb loses some of its qualities. It is possible to keep fresh herbs for about two weeks in the refrigerator. Make sure they are completely dry and pack them in airtight containers. The usual plastic airtight boxes are quite suitable.

However fresh herbs are often not available but dried herbs are a more than adequate second-best. As mentioned earlier, you can buy these in a shop, but you will be more able to control their quality and age if you pick and dry them yourself. Pick herbs on a dry, sunny morning, making sure that all the dew has evaporated. Try not to damage the plant more than necessary and do not bruise the leaves.

If the leaves are the part of the plant that is to be used (for example, thyme or rosemary) they should be harvested when the plant is just coming into flower. If the flower is to be used (for example, camomile or lavender) it should be picked in full bloom. It is said that herbs picked when the moon is waning have less sap in their leaves and stalks and will dry better. Herbs to be used fresh should be gathered when the moon is waxing. Roots are also then at their softest and are easier to pull up after it has rained when the ground is soft. Most roots are best harvested in the autumn.

Find a warm dry place, out of the sun, to dry the herbs. Spread them out on a piece of paper and let them dry slowly. You can stretch a piece of muslin over them to keep off the dust but make sure the air can circulate freely. You can also hang them up in little bunches with their heads downward. If the weather is very cold or damp they can be dried in a very slow oven. Roots must be cut lengthwise to quicken the drying process.

Store the herbs in airtight jars, pots or tins, but do protect them from the light. However attractive a herb rack with rows of glass jars may look, it is not suitable for storing herbs if you want to keep them at their best. Store them instead in a cool, dark, dry cupboard and they will retain their maximum aroma and quality. There are many different opinions about how long dried herbs will keep. I would only say buy or dry small quantities at a time and, if possible, renew once a year.

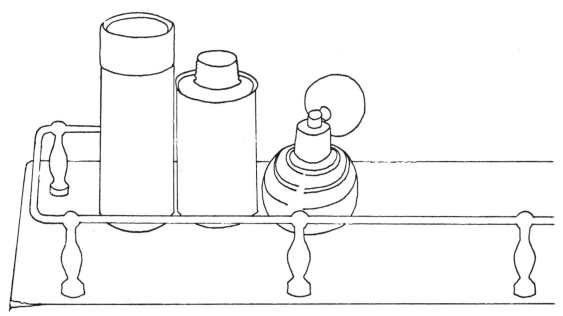

3 HOW TO PREPARE HERBS

There are various methods of preparing herbs for use in lotions and creams. The recipes in this book involve five basic herbal preparations:

a. Infusions

This is like making herbal tea. Pour boiling water over the herb (fresh or dried) and leave it for about 5 minutes. Then sieve. As when making ordinary tea, warm the pot first and ensure that it has a well-fitting lid. None of the aromatic substances should be lost. Infusions are suitable for tender plants whose active ingredients are readily imparted to the liquid.

b. Cold Infusions

Here the herb must be allowed to steep in a cold liquid. The time this takes depends on the herb used. The process must take place in a hermetically-sealed airtight pot, and wine or alcohol are usually used. Herbal vinegars are also prepared in this way.

c. Decoctions

By this method the herb is boiled, usually for about 15 minutes, again, depending on the herb used. Decoctions are usually prepared from the hard parts of plants, like roots or tree bark.

d. Essential Oils

In preparing herbal creams essential oils are the most effective way of adding herbs. Take ½ cup of fresh crushed herbs (or 2 dessertspoonfuls of dried herbs) to ½ litre of vegetable oil. Almond oil is the most suitable for use in cosmetics but sunflower oil will do very well and is cheaper. Add 1 tablespoon of white wine vinegar. Pour the mixture into a screw-topped jar and shake vigorously. Put this in a warm light place, preferably in the sun. Let the oil mature for three weeks. Strain well and pour it into a suitable bottle. If you think the aroma is not strong enough, you can pour the strained oil over a fresh lot of herbs and repeat the process.

e. Tinctures

This is a simple tincture made by pounding 100 grams of dried herb into a powder and adding 1 litre of medicinal alcohol. Keep this for two weeks in a screw-topped jar or bottle in a warm place. Shake the container daily. Filter the tincture through a coffee filter before using it.

NB When water is called for, always use distilled water as hard water is bad for your skin. The soft continental mineral waters such as Perrier water can be used if they are available.

4 USING HERBS IN COSMETICS

This book is intended as a basis for you to develop your own personal creams and lotions. You can do this by choosing one of the herbs or fruits mentioned in this chapter and adding it, in the form of a herbal infusion, or tincture or essential oil, to one of the basic formulae given for creams and lotions later in the book.

Choose the herb which is most suitable for your hair or skin type, and most easily obtainable. Then choose a cream or lotion and replace the simple oil by an equal quantity of essential oil of herb. Distilled water or rosewater can be replaced by an equal quantity of herbal infusion. In the case of hair tonics, the alcohol ingredient may be replaced by the same amount of herbal tincture.

To help you decide where herbal substitutes can be used there is an asterisk in the formulae next to the ingredients which can be replaced by herbal substances. For example, in the recipe for Sweet Almond Oil Cream on page 17, the almond oil may be replaced by an essential oil of herb (like camomile oil), *or* the rosewater can be replaced by a herbal infusion.

Another way of adding herbs to cosmetics is to pound a quantity of fresh herb directly into your creams. This has to be done very thoroughly and requires a lot of energy! A pestle and mortar are essential for this. It is also possible to add plant or fruit juices directly to the creams and lotions. This is most easily done in a liquidiser.

The following guide will help you decide which herbs are most suitable for your particular skin or hair type:

1. ASTRINGENT HERBS

The most important of these are plantain, lemon, hazel and bilberry. Witch hazel has also very important astringent properties but this is usually bought directly from a chemist in the form of witch hazel (or *hamamelis*) water.

a. **Plantain**
Many people who think of plantain as a common weed will be surprised to hear that it is a very valuable herb. Its astringent properties will help to close open pores and refine a coarse skin. The juice of the fresh herb can be directly incorporated into creams, milks and lotions. Infusions and essential oils are also easily prepared from it.

b. **Lemon**
This must be one of the best known cosmetic plants. It has a mild astringent and tonic effect on the skin. It will also lighten and freshen the complexion. This is particularly useful in winter when you are faced with a yellowish faded tan. A small quantity of lemon juice added to creams will also help to soothe an irritated skin.

c. **Hazel**
In this book it is the hazel leaves rather than the nuts which we are concerned with. These are astringent and will help to close open pores. Use a little fresh sap, or prepare an essential oil or infusion.

d. **Bilberry**
Both the berries and the leaves of this plant have astringent properties. However, it is the leaves which are usually used. The blue colouring in the berries makes them more

13

appropriate for ancient Britons than for twentieth-century man or woman. Bilberry leaves are recommended for use in anti-wrinkle creams. Prepare an essential oil or infusion.

2. HERBS FOR SOFTENING AND MOISTURISING THE SKIN

a. Marsh-mallow
This is the most valuable herb in this group as the roots contain a viscous substance which is a well known emollient (softener). It can be extracted by steeping the finely chopped root in cold water. The liquid will become gelatinous and when sieved it can be added to lotions and creams. Common mallow and musk mallow can be used in the same way, but their roots do not contain as much of the emollient substances as those of the marsh-mallow.

b. Cucumber
The juice of this fruit also has a moisturising and soothing effect on the skin. It will lighten and freshen the complexion. People with over-sensitive skin will find cucumber a particularly valuable plant.

c. Camomile
An emollient plant which grows along every country lane. This herb can be used in the usual ways but a very valuable camomile oil can also be prepared with 100 grams fresh camomile flowers and 1 litre sunflower oil. Put the flowers and oil into a bowl and stand it for 3 hours in a pan of boiling water 'au bain marie' (or in the top of a double boiler). Press out

the oil from the camomile flowers and filter it through a coffee filter. This oil can be added to cold creams, using one part oil to five parts cold cream. It can also be used directly on the skin to soften particularly rough patches. Camomile is especially recommended for a coarse rough skin.

3. OTHER HERBS FOR SKIN CREAMS AND LOTIONS

a. Coltsfoot
This common weed will soften the skin, but it also has mild astringent and antiseptic qualities. Add the juice or prepare an infusion of the leaves or flowers to add to creams and tonics. Coltsfoot will tone up a flabby skin and is also used in anti-acne mixtures.

b. Marigold
Marigold flowers will tone up the skin and are strongly antiseptic. The essential oil can be added to cold creams or used directly to heal minor cuts, grazes and pimples. A very simple, if not completely natural, marigold cream can be made by adding 5 or 6 chopped marigold heads to the contents of a jar of vaseline. Warm this gently in the top of a double boiler for about 1—2 hours. The resulting cream should then be sieved and poured into pots. It will have a deep golden colour. Marigold infusions can also be used.

c. St John's wort
In Germany this is considered to be the miracle-worker of the cosmetic herbs. Take 500 grams

of the flowering tops of the plant and chop them finely. Add 1 litre of sunflower oil and ½ litre of white wine. Mix well and leave it to stand for 3 days. Then warm it in a double saucepan until the wine has evaporated. The oil obtained will heal a damaged skin and soothe irritations. It will also help to cure heat rashes. It should be added to creams and lotions in the ratio 1:5.

However, *never go out into the sun after using it* because some pigmentation of the skin can result. It is advisable to use this oil, or recipes containing it, only before going to bed at night. Next morning wash your face and all will be well. St John's wort oil can be bought ready prepared in some health food shops or prepare an essential oil as described on page 12. A few drops of this oil in the ear can also help to soothe earache.

4. HERBS FOR HAIR

Infusions or cold infusions in alcohol of yarrow, rosemary, stinging nettle, horsetail and chillies can all be added to hair waters and lotions. These herbs are all used to help prevent seborrhoea. Rosemary, nettles and chillies are also said to stimulate the blood circulation in the scalp and to encourage hair growth.

5 FACE CREAMS

The use of face creams to protect and nourish the skin has been known since the ancient Chinese civilisations. However the first really useful recipe, which still serves as the basis of most cold creams, is that of the Greek doctor Galen (his formula follows in the recipes).

In the Middle Ages such refinements were rarely used, and instead herbs were simmered in lard or butter to make medical and beauty ointments. Butter still makes an acceptable face cream for those with a very dry skin, but lard will enlarge the pores and is hardly a fragrant base for cosmetics.

Later the making of face creams became more sophisticated but some extraordinary cosmetics were developed such as 'Fucus of Cosmetick of River Crabs', described by William Salmon in his *Polygraphices* 1685:

Take of the flesh which remains in the extremities of the great claws of river Crabs (being boiled) a sufficient quantity, which dry gently and then extract a deep tincture with rectified spirit of wine; evaporate part of the menstruum, till the tincture have a good thickness or body; with which (the skin being cleansed) anoint the cheeks first applying over it some albifying Cosmetick.

In 1640 John Parkinson described another beauty cream made from lupins which would take away all marks of smallpox and make the lady 'look more amiable'. Ladies do therefore 'use the meale of lupins mingled with the gall of a goate and some juyce of lemons to make into the forme of a soft ointment'.

Gall of goats and claws of river crabs are not easy to obtain these days. The recipes that follow should cause fewer problems.

All the creams are easy to make and require no complicated implements. An electric mixer is useful and it cuts down the time needed to beat the ingredients together, but it is not essential.

It is important to have the ingredients at the same temperature to facilitate the blending of the water with the oils and fats.

Always add the watery ingredients drop by drop to the oils and fats in the same way that you would add the oil to the egg yolks when making mayonnaise.

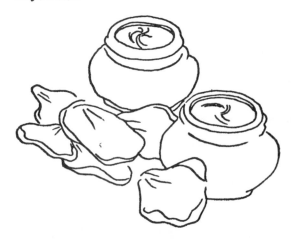

Not all these creams contain a preservative (the alcohol or spirit ingredient). If you want to make larger quantities or keep these for some time, outside a refrigerator, you can buy chemical preservatives from the chemist.

All these face creams can serve as a basis for the herbs described in the previous chapter. Almond oil can always be replaced by the cheaper sunflower oil.

Don't be too put off by the exact measures. A little experience will soon have you using teaspoons and dessertspoons instead of grams and you will soon learn to adjust the texture of your creams by using a few flakes more or less of white wax. However, it is easier to have the exact measures to begin with.

GALEN'S COLD CREAM

150g.   White wax
400g.   Sweet almond oil *
1 cup   Distilled water with a few drops of spirit vinegar *

This recipe, which was invented by Galen in the second century *AD*, is always thought of as the original formula for cold cream. He melted together the oil and wax and then added the water and spirit. Instead of almond oil, however, Galen used oil of roses — a substance far too precious and expensive for everyday use nowadays. You can, however, use rosewater instead of distilled water, and you can perfume the cream with a little lavender or rosemary extract. It makes an excellent base cream for all but the most greasy skin. Astringent or emollient herb extract can be added, *or* prepare an essential oil with the almond oil, *or* a herbal infusion with the distilled water.

The following five recipes are for creams suitable for dry to normal skins.

ALMOND OIL CREAM

40g.   Sweet almond oil *
10g.   White wax
40g.   Rosewater *

Melt the oils and fats together. Add the rosewater slowly, beating well. You can prepare an essential oil with the almond oil *or* replace the rosewater with a herbal infusion.

COLD CREAM WITH PEANUT AND CASTOR OILS

8g.   White wax
10g.   Spermaceti
55g.   Peanut oil *
20g.   Distilled water *
5g.   Castor oil

Melt fats and oils together. Beat in distilled water. Peanut oil or distilled water can be used as a herbal base. This is an excellent cream for very dry skin.

HONEY CREAM

1 dessertspoon   Honey
A few drops   Almond oil*
1   Egg white

Beat the egg white until stiff, then gradually add the oil and honey. Go on beating until a thick smooth cream is prepared. This simple kitchen recipe will feed all types of skin. For a very dry skin a little more almond oil can be added. The cream can't be kept for much longer than a week in the refrigerator and it is rather sticky to use. However, if you feel your skin is a little out of condition and you have an egg white left over it is worth preparing and you can then give your skin a week's 'cure'. An essential oil can, of course, be prepared to replace the almond oil, but, in this case, (and you'll only be using it for a week) it is not so important. The important ingredients of this cream are the egg white and honey.

17

NOURISHING FACE CREAM WITH SESAME OIL

5g.   White wax
10g.   Lanolin
10g.   Spermaceti
50g.   Sesame oil
25g.   Rosewater *

Melt the oils and fats together and then (as usual) beat in the water. An excellent cream for dry or undernourished skin. Rosewater can be replaced by a herbal infusion.

ORANGE BLOSSOM FACE CREAM

4g.   White wax
20g.   Almond oil
2g.   Spermaceti
10g.   Orange blossom infusion

Again oils and fats must be melted together and then the orange blossom infusion added. Orange blossom is fragrant, mildly astringent and will tone up the skin and freshen the complexion. It can be replaced by another herbal infusion if preferred.

A FAT-FREE CREAM FOR AN OILY SKIN

1 coffeespoon Natural pectin powder
30g.   Alcohol *
15g.   Glycerine
45g.   Rosewater *

Moisten the pectin powder with a little alcohol. Then mix this gradually with the glycerine and the rest of the alcohol. Add the rosewater. Heat this mixture slowly until it boils. Let it boil for 3—4 minutes, then pour it into a jar where it will form a jelly. Herbs can be added in an infusion instead of the rosewater, or in a cold infusion prepared with the alcohol.

An Incomparable Cosmetick of Pearl

Dissolve Pearls in juyce of lemons or distilled vinegar, which digest in Horse-dung, till they send forth a clear oil which will swim on the top, this is one of the most excellent Cosmeticks or Beautifiers in the world; this oil if well prepared is richly worth seven pound an ounce.

William Salmon, *Polygraphices*, 1685

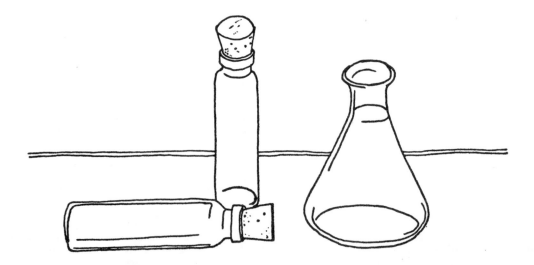

6 SKIN TONICS

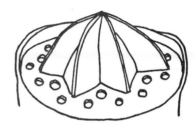

Skin tonics are used to remove excess oil from the skin. They are refreshing, stimulating and will tone up the complexion. Tonics are often used after a cleansing lotion to remove the last traces of dirt and grease from the face but they can also be used by themselves to clean the face or, when the skin is very greasy, after washing with soap and water.

WITCH HAZEL AND ROSEWATER TONIC

This is the simplest and one of the best skin tonics. It is very well known and any chemist will make it up for you. But it is just as easy to make it yourself by mixing 2 parts rosewater to 1 part witch hazel. These proportions are for a normal to greasy skin. Those with a very oily skin can increase the proportion of witch hazel and those with drier skin should increase the proportion of rosewater.

Astringent Skin Tonics

These tonics all contain alcohol and are not suitable for people with very dry or sensitive skins. Instead they should use the simple herbal lotions described in the next chapter. All the tonics in this chapter are based on herbal or vegetable ingredients and need no additions.

ORANGE AND LEMON TONIC

3   Lemons
1   Cucumber
1   Orange
3   dessertspoons Rosewater
30g. Alcohol

Extract the juice from the orange, lemons and cucumber and mix this with the other ingredients. This makes a potent lotion, good for skin colour and for those who suffer from blackheads.

CUCUMBER TONIC

1 Cucumber
Elderflowers
Distilled water
Brandy

Peel the cucumber and slice thinly. Put it into a pan and add enough water to cover it. Simmer until the cucumber is soft. Mash it and put in a muslin cloth to drip. Press as much of the juice through the cloth as you can. Add 1 part brandy to 2 parts cucumber juice. Prepare an elderflower infusion with 3 flowers to ¼ litre distilled water. Add 1 part elderflower infusion to 2 parts cucumber and brandy mixture. This makes an excellent lotion to clear a troubled skin.

STIMULATING TONIC

5g.	Glycerine
40g.	Rosewater
40g.	Orange blossom infusion
40g.	Distilled water
40g.	Witch hazel
10g.	Cherry laurel water
5g.	Alcohol
20g.	Eau de Cologne

This tonic is obviously more trouble to prepare, but if you have a dull, flabby skin it is worthwhile. Cherry laurel water can be bought at chemists' shops but it is also possible to prepare a strong decoction from the fresh leaves of the plant (*prunus Laurocerasus*) by boiling a handful of chopped leaves in ¼ litre distilled water for 15—20 minutes. Filter the liquid through a coffee filter, add it to the other ingredients in a screw-topped jar or bottle and shake the mixture vigorously.

ORANGE BLOSSOM TONIC

60g.	Orange blossom infusion
35g.	Alcohol
2g.	Glycerine

Prepare the infusion with 1 dessertspoonful dried orange blossom to ¼ litre distilled water. Filter this well and shake it together with the other ingredients. A simple and soothing mixture.

ROSEMARY TONIC

1 small bunch	Rosemary
¼ litre	Distilled water
½ measure	Brandy

Simmer the bunch of fresh rosemary in the mixture of distilled water and brandy for 20 minutes. Filter this mixture and you have an excellent mild face tonic.

Rosemary is one of the most loved of herbs and references to it can be found in many old writings. Anne of Cleves wore it in a wreath at her wedding. Elizabeth of Hungary was said to keep her skin free from wrinkles by using it in her face lotion, and Sir Thomas More was happy to let it 'runne all over my garden walls ... because it is a herb sacred to remembrance, and therefore to friendship.'

In 1655, in *The Queen's Closet Opened*, W.M., Queen Henrietta Maria's cook, wrote this:
'To Make the Face Fair and for a Stinking Breathe — Take the flowers of rosemary, and seethe them in white wine, with which wash your face; if you drink Thereof it will make you have a sweet breathe.'

7 COMPLEXION LOTIONS

These simple herbal lotions are the easiest way to apply herbs to your complexion. They will not cleanse a really oily skin but they can be used after cleansing or washing the face to clear an impure skin or improve the complexion colour and texture.

Those with sensitive skins will find some of these lotions invaluable and can use them to clean the face, with a piece of cotton wool, if they do this regularly and thoroughly.

Some of these lotions are made with the most common kitchen vegetables, and others with way-side herbs or garden flowers. But don't neglect the most prosaic ones. They are often the most effective.

An impure and troubled skin can often be cleared by regularly rinsing the face with decoctions of white or savoy CABBAGE.

YARROW decoction will help to remove black-heads, but rinse your face well after using this herb and apply a good simple cold cream as yarrow can sometimes irritate the skin.

Infusions of LOVAGE and VERBENA will help to keep the skin free from impurities, as will an infusion made from BORAGE leaves and flowers.

CAMOMILE infusion is invaluable to clean sensitive skins and will soften and smooth a rough irritated complexion.

BALM infusion, usually drunk for its tranquillising qualities, will also soothe and soften skin irritations.

SPEEDWELL is said to benefit those with itching eczema.

ORANGE BLOSSOM infusion makes not only a delicious and refreshing tea, but can also serve as a complexion rinse. It is also an ingredient in the skin tonics as it will tone up a pale flabby skin and close pores.

MARSH-MALLOW is, as we have already seen, well known for its emollient qualities and it is highly recommended for sensitive skins easily irritated by hard (lime-containing) water. Make a decoction by putting 5—10 grams of marsh-mallow root in 1 litre of cold water. Bring the water to the boil and let it simmer for 10—15 minutes.

One of the better known complexion lotions can be made with citrus peel. Carefully peel LEMONS, ORANGES, GRAPEFRUIT so that you do not have too much pith. Put the peel into 4 times their volume of cold distilled water. Leave this to stand overnight. Next morning filter this mixture carefully and put it in a bottle and keep it in the fridge. Use cotton wool to apply the liquid to your face twice daily. It will stimulate the complexion and clear the skin.

To lighten your complexion colour there is an ancient recipe using an infusion of ELDERBERRIES, WHITE CLOVER and DAISIES. It is also said to remove freckles.

Another flower lotion is made from ROSE and LILY petals. Let a handful of petals steep in cold water for an hour. Bring the liquid to the boil and then let it simmer for an hour. Cool and sieve. This fragrant water will soften the skin and improve the complexion tone.

MARIGOLD petals can be infused to make a lightly disinfectant astringent lotion for an oily skin and DAISY water is an old folk remedy which will help to clear up spots and pimples.

More prosaic is CHICKWEED which is said to refine a coarse skin and improve the skin texture.

For a light astringent lotion without alcohol prepare a decoction of equal amounts of THYME, ROSEMARY, and HAWTHORN and BLACK-BERRY leaves; use this daily. It will keep in the refrigerator for at least a week.

To make a lady fair

Take two pair of Calves feet, boil them in 9 quarts of water till half be consumed, then put to them one pound of rice, boil it with crums of white bread steep'd before in milk, add two pounds of fresh butter, 10 whites of eggs and their shells, then distill all together putting in a little comfrey and alum of the rock and wash with it.
    Richard Pynsens, *A Proper New Book of Cookerie*, 1576

To delay heat and cleare the face

Take 3 pintes of conduit water, boyle therein 2 ounces of French barley, change your water and put in the barley again. Repeate this so long till your water purchase no colour from the barley, but become very cleare. Boyle the last three pintes to a quart then mixe halfe a pinte of white wine therein, and when it is cold, wring the juyce of two or three good lemmins therein, and use the same for the Morpheuse, heat of the face or hands and to cleare the skinne.
    Sir Hugh Platt, *Delights for Ladies*, 1609

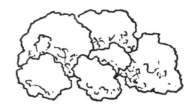

8 CLEANSING METHODS

Cleansing creams and milks are, of course, exactly what they say, methods of cleansing the skin without using soap and water. And indeed for those with dry sensitive skin, easily irritated by astringent products, they are very useful. There are, however, other ways of cleansing your face, and for most people soap and water does very well. The cosmetic industry may have persuaded them otherwise but a mild unperfumed soap (like baby soap) and soft water is ideal for the majority of people. If you live in an area where the water is hard (lime-containing) it is advisable to keep a bottle of distilled, soft mineral water, or, even better, rainwater to wash your face with. Rainwater is obviously the cheapest of these and it is also ideal for washing your hair. So if you have a garden or balcony do all you can to find an old-fashioned rainwater barrel or some other container to catch this valuable cosmetic substance.

In periods of prolonged drought you can give your complexion a luxury wash in lukewarm MILK or even better BUTTERMILK.

CUCUMBER is another ideal cleanser for the normal to oily skin: mix a little cucumber purée with ¼ litre milk and keep this in the refrigerator. You can use it in the same way as a conventional cleansing cream, but shake it before use. You will, of course, have to renew the mixture twice a week. With a little more trouble you can make this cucumber-milk cleanser which will keep for a week in the refrigerator: grate ½ cucumber in ¼ litre milk; boil this for 5 minutes and then cool, sieve and bottle it. The simplest cucumber cleanser is to keep the cucumber skin left over from a salad and carefully wipe your face with the inside of it. Those who usually wash with soap and water can give their complexion a refreshing tone-up on salad days.

Removing eye make-up is one thing that soap and water certainly cannot do so keep a small bottle of SWEET ALMOND OIL in the bathroom. While using it to remove your eye make-up you will also nourish the delicate skin around your eyes. Extremely dry skin can be cleansed by using almond oil and removing the excess oil with camomile infusion.

ROSEWATER is also a useful cleanser. This can be bought ready-made or prepared from fresh rose petals.

Less fragrant but very effective is the use of OAT-MEAL. Dampen this and use it gently as a sponge. It is an excellent dirt remover and will help to clear blackheads.

GROUND ALMONDS can also make an effective cleansing cream: mix 1 dessertspoon ground almonds with just enough rosewater to make it liquid. It should have a 'pea soup' texture. Apply this to the face with cotton wool and rinse off with a herbal lotion or soft water.

These simple lotions and the recipes that follow will not be enough to remove heavy make-up. It is hardly necessary to point out that regular use of heavy make-up damages the complexion but, if you do use it, cold cream (page 17) makes an ideal remover.

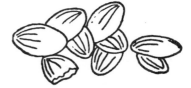

ALMOND MILK

50g	Peeled sweet almonds
50g	Caster sugar
90g.	Distilled water

With a pestle and mortar crush the almonds with the sugar and a little water. Add the rest of the water and let it stand for 1—2 hours. Sieve through a piece of muslin and press out all the liquid. This is an old French beauty milk which will give the skin a velvety feel. Chemical preservative may be added.

ALMOND CREAM

12 dessertspoons	Sweet almond oil
2 teaspoons	Butter
2 teaspoons	Rosewater *
2 teaspoons	Grated castile soap

Melt the soap and oil together in a double saucepan. Gradually add the butter and rosewater while beating vigorously. Take from the heat but continue beating until the cream is cooled.

VASELINE CREAM

15g.	Beeswax
14g.	White vaseline
50g.	Almond oil *
20g.	Rosewater *

This is not a completely natural cream but it is a useful cleanser and makes a good base for herbal oil *or* infusion. Bring the beeswax and vaseline in one container, and the rosewater and oil in two further containers, to the same temperature (10⁰ Centigrade, 50⁰ Fahrenheit). Remove from the heat and add the rosewater and oil to the vaseline and beeswax mixture, beating all the time. **24** Continue beating until cool.

COCONUT BUTTER CREAM

150g.	Coconut butter
50g.	Almond oil
100g.	Distilled water *

Warm the coconut butter until it melts. Gradually add warm almond oil and water, beating all the time. Remove from the heat. Continue beating until cool.

VIOLET MILK

¼ litre milk
2 dessertspoons sweet violets

Boil the milk and then let it cool for a few minutes. Pour the warm milk over the flowers and leave it to stand for 2 hours. Sieve and keep the milk in the refrigerator (it will keep for about a week). Clean your face with cotton wool dipped into the milk every morning and evening. This can be used as a Spring clean for the complexion, which often becomes greyish and dulled in the winter.

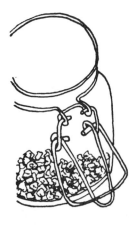

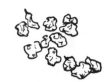

Balles for the Face

*Take greate Allecant reusons [raisins] a quarter of
a pounde, stone them but wash them not and beat
them in a mortar very fine, take as many almonds,
not jordans, but of the common sort and blanck
them and drye them in a cloth well and beate
them in a stone mortar also very fine, when you
have done this to them bothe, mingle them bothe
together and beate them againe, and put to it half
a quarter of a pounde of browne leavened bread,
wheaten bread, and beate them altogether and
mingle them well together and then take it and
make it in little balles and then wash your face at
night with one of them in rayne water. If you will
have this only to wash your hands, put in a little
Venice soape but put none of that in for youre
face.*

   Mary Fairfax, *Still-room Book*, 1630.

A recipe still worth trying if you have the time.

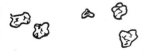

9 PIMPLES, SPOTS AND ACNE

This is an unattractive title for a chapter, but of all beauty problems it is perhaps spottiness which causes the greatest unhappiness. For serious skin diseases it is of course necessary to go to a doctor but everyone has periods of skin eruptions, particularly during adolescence, and for these there are herbal drinks and natural remedies which can often be used successfully.

The most important aspect of skin care is diet. A balanced diet, containing enough fresh vegetables, fruit, low fat yogurts and plenty of whole grain products, should ensure that the condition of both skin and hair is as good as possible. No one can look their best on a fatty diet and vast quantities of sweet and starchy food, even if they do manage to stay slim.

Another frequent cause of spots and pimples is an over-oily skin. This can be alleviated by frequent and thorough cleansing of the skin, and the application of astringent skin tonics (see Chapter 6). It is possible to add a little CARROT juice or COLTSFOOT tincture to Rosemary Tonic or Orange and Lemon Tonic for mild cases of acne.

Herbalists also pay a great deal of attention to 'depuratives' — those herbs which serve to purify the system. These are taken internally and while cleaning you inside will purify the blood and help to ensure a clear skin on the outside. Many of these herbs are included in the 'Spring cures' intended to tone up a sluggish system and purify the body, and therefore the skin, after the long dark winter. These herbs include STINGING NETTLES, CHICKWEED, BETONY, SHEPHERD'S PURSE, BORAGE, BIRCH leaves, PLANTAIN, BURDOCK and WATERCRESS.

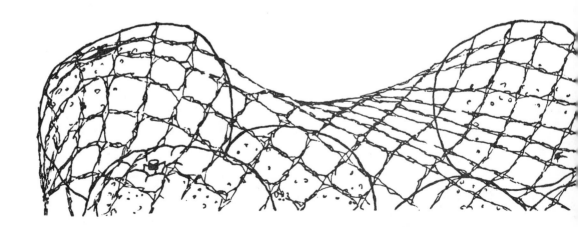

The young leaves, shoots and even roots of these plants can be used to make herbal infusions. Young nettles can be cooked and eaten like SPINACH (itself a good depurative) or used in soups with a few plantain tops and a little chickweed or shepherd's purse. Depurative salads can be made including the first spinach leaves, a few young DANDELION leaves, watercress and a little SAVORY, LOVAGE and borage.

Simple herbal teas can also be effective. Birch leaf tea is a particularly good cure for acne: drink one cup before breakfast every morning. Betony can be used in the same way for people who have a tendency to eczema. Dried burdock root is available all the year and will help to clear a spotty skin. It is prepared as a decoction, 40—60 grams to a litre of water. Drink a wine glass of this after every meal. It can also be used externally as a lotion. Another face lotion can be prepared by infusing ELDER leaves and adding 1 teaspoon HONEY to every ½ litre of infusion. Use this daily. SPEEDWELL, savory and PENNYWORT infusions are also useful face lotions to purify the skin and they make effective compresses (see Chapter 15) for use if the outbreaks are more widespread. Carrot juice compresses will also help clear up spots and acne.

For that odd distressing pimple it isn't even necessary to go to the trouble of making an infusion, squeeze some juice from a MISTLETOE berry directly onto it, or a little of the sap found in dandelion stems. This last will help to heal the spot but it does make a black mark on the skin temporarily so it is better to put it on at night.

That attractive little plant with the consoling name of SELF HEAL will also help to clear up a difficult spot. Crush one of the leaves and apply directly to the infected area. If it is a recurring sore you can stick the leaf onto the face with a piece of sticking plaster overnight. My son had a very unsightly cold sore which regularly reappeared on the same place; one application of self heal and it never returned.

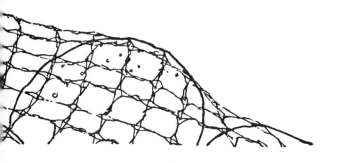

DEPURATIVE HERBAL TEA: (a)

20g. White dead-nettle
20g. Juniper berries
20g. Burdock root
20g. Stinging nettle
20g. Meadowsweet

Mix the herbs well together. Prepare an infusion with 2 teaspoons herbal mixture to ½ litre water. Drink 1 cup mornings and evenings.

DEPURATIVE HERBAL TEA: (b)

Lavender
White clover
Marigold petals
Soft inner bark of beech or elder

Mix these together in equal quantities and prepare an infusion as in the previous recipe. This is an old Balkan remedy recommended by David Conway in *The Magic of Herbs.*

DEPURATIVE HERBAL TEA: (c)

15g. Sage
20g. Raspberry leaves
20g. Hawthorn leaves

Boil 3 soupspoons of this herbal mixture in 1 litre of water. Let it reduce to about ¾ litre. Drink 1 cup daily.

DEPURATIVE HERBAL TEA: (d)

Meadowsweet
Mugwort
Hawthorn leaves
Borage flowers

Mix these herbs in equal quantities and use 2 dessertspoons to ¾ litre water. Bring to the boil and simmer for one minute. Drink 3 cups daily.

PURIFYING JUICE

Borage
Watercress
Dandelion

Take equal quantities of these herbs and extract the juice in a liquidiser. Take 1 teaspoonful twice daily. You can keep this in the deep freeze.

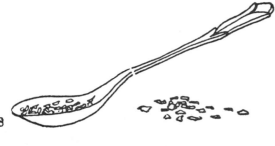

Of Primroses and Cowslips

The juice of these flowers is commended to cleanse the spots or marks of the face, whereof some genlewoman have found good experience.
John Parkinson, *Paradisi in Sole Paradisius Terrestris*, 1629.

FACE LOTION

25g.	Alcohol
5g.	Rosewater
5g.	Lemon oil
2 drops Bergamot	

Shake the ingredients together in a jar or bottle.

This astringent lotion will help to clear spots and blackheads which are the result of an over-oily skin. Wash the skin daily with this lotion.

Skin problems were obviously just as worrying in the eighteenth century as can be seen in this truly extraordinary recipe. To try this you must have been desperate and even then I'm afraid it did a lot more harm than good:

Water of White Melon to Make the Skin Pure

Take white melons whose skins are well cleaned. Cut these in pieces as thick as a finger. Throw away the middle part. Then take of the following. Allum four ounces, quicksilver which is dead, rock allum burnt, each an ounce. Hog's fat two ounces, terpentine 1 pound, twelve eggs crusted with their shells. Lemon soup as much as you like. Sugar 40 ounces, Goatsmilk and white wine each one pint. Put this altogether in a glass. Distill this over a soft fire, it is most agreeable to wash with.
Simon Witgeest, 1715

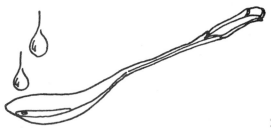

10 SKIN AND SUN

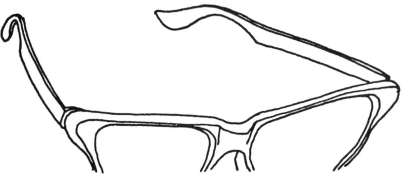

A few years ago a British dermatologist compared the skin of a baby's bottom to that of an 80-year-old man. The difference was minimal. Samples taken from the back of the hand however told another story. The contrast there was striking. The reason for this was clear: bottoms seldom see the sun whereas a hand is constantly exposed to it. Sun ages the skin. If you want to stay young and beautiful you'll have to be pale and interesting. But fashion has for many years dictated otherwise and most of us are not prepared to forego the pleasures of sand, sea and sunbathing.

There are many products which will reduce the damage caused by sun on skin, and it is not necessarily the most expensive of these which are the most effective. Natural oils can also be used and these are generally much cheaper than ready-made sun oils. Both OLIVE OIL and COCONUT OIL absorb ultra-violet rays and will help to ensure an even tan. For people with very sensitive, easily burnt skin SESAME OIL will provide an almost total screen. These oils can be mixed together and perfumed as described in the recipes on the following pages. But these oil-based lotions have one major disadvantage: they are rather sticky. In the garden or on shingle beaches this is not so important but on a sandy beach it can be most uncomfortable. On the other hand these oils will not wash off so easily if you go for a swim, and it is generally agreed that salt water on an unprotected skin is the cause of the most painful sunburn. A less greasy sun tan lotion is the usual vinaigrette dressing (without the garlic and seasoning): an oil and vinegar mixture promotes a splendid, if rather smelly, sun tan.

CARROTS are another kitchen remedy for sunburn. It is said that if you eat raw carrots before sunbathing you will not be so badly burnt. There is some scientific truth in this 'old wives tale' and it is certainly more desirable than the anti-sunburn tablets which have recently achieved some popularity. It is also said that if you eat enough carrots your skin will become yellowish brown without any sun! But this can be dangerous. In 1975 a Belgian carrot addict died from an overdose of carrots. It transpired that he never ate anything else.

There are, of course, many curious remedies to be found in the old herbals. One sixteenth-century lotion described by Sir Hugh Platt was only applicable to babies:

'Wash the face and body of a sucking child with breast milke, or cowe milke mixed with water, every night and the childes skinne will wax cleare and resist sunburning.'

But the Anglo-Saxon *Leech Book of Bald* described something very similar to our oil and vinegar mixture:

'That all the body maybe of a clear and glad and bright hue, take oil and dregs of old wine equally much, put them in a mortar, mingle well together and smear the body with this in the sun.'

If, in spite of everything, you do suffer sunburn, there are several effective herbal cures. Infusions of ELDER flowers or WHITE DEAD-NETTLE are very soothing. A few CAMOMILE flowers boiled gently in ¼ litre milk will also cool and soften a sun-damaged skin. If you have a QUINCE tree anywhere in your vicinity it is worth making quince pip emollient: using 2 parts water to 1 part pips crush the quince pips, cover with water and leave to stand, stirring occasionally; when a gelatinous substance is formed the emollient is ready. Sieve it and apply to the damaged skin. This can also be added to face creams to soothe skin irritations. WHITE WINE or BUTTERMILK compresses will also neutralise the effects of excessive sunbathing.

LAVENDER SUN OIL

40g.	Coconut oil
40g.	Olive oil
5g.	Essential oil of lavender

Shake together.

SUN OIL FOR SENSITIVE SKINS

60g.	Sesame oil
35g.	Olive oil
A few drops	Bergamot oil

Shake together.

DEEP TAN SUN OIL

30g.	Coconut oil
30g.	Cocoa butter
A few drops	Bergamot oil

Melt the coconut oil and cocoa butter together. Remove from the heat and add Bergamot oil. Beat until cool.

To Soothe Sunburn:

For sunburn boil in butter tender ivy twigs, smear therewith.
    The Leech Book of Bald   **31**

11 WRINKLES

There are no cosmetic wonders which can prevent the skin becoming wrinkled. Wrinkles come with age and no one has yet discovered the secret of everlasting youth. It is possible nowadays to have a surgical face lift, at great expense, but the unnaturally expressionless mask which this produces is rarely attractive. Moreover, in some cases, the effect is short-lived and in any case it is not a permanent solution. Wrinkles are not ugly and it is sad when people (and women are by no means the only ones to undergo regular face lifts) are so desperately eager to recapture their lost youth. However, premature wrinkles can be depressing. No one aged forty wants to look fifty! The most successful and natural way to prevent this happening is regular face massage. With a little practice this is quite easy to do yourself.

FACE MASSAGE

If you have a dry to normal skin use cold cream to massage your face. People with oilier skins can use cold creams prepared with witch hazel rather than rosewater, or they can sprinkle a little baby powder on their hands.

First, cleanse your face thoroughly of all make-up. Wash your hands. Wash your face with warm water and gently pat it dry. Cream or powder your hands. Then:

1. With the palms of your hands stroke your forehead gently from one temple to another.
2. Use the same movement from chin to temples.
3. Stroke from the corners of the jawbone to the neck and shoulders.
4. Stroke gently around the eyes, starting at the nose and continuing to the eyebrows.
5. Repeat the first four movements more firmly, but don't press hard.
6. Rub gently with the fingertips in a spiral movement in the same places and in the same directions.
7. Where wrinkles are forming, very gently and gradually pinch the skin between thumb and forefinger, and press gradually at the same time with middle and ring fingers.
8. Gently beat against the same places with fore and middle fingers. Gradually increase the tempo and bring the ring finger and little finger into action.
9. Continue very gently beating all the fingers over the face in the same way as you would drum them on the edge of a table. Slowly increase speed and pressure and then return to your original tempo.

This massage takes a little time to perfect but it will tone up the underlying face muscles and improve the elasticity of the skin.

To prevent wrinkling of the delicate skin round the eyes use ALMOND OIL to remove eye make-up and wipe it from the nose to the ears. There are several herbs which are reputed to help prevent wrinkles and these can be added to cold creams or applied as infusions. PRIMROSES or COWSLIPS are often used to this end, probably because of the 'doctrine of signatures' whereby a plant which resembles a certain part of the body was thought to cure it. If you examine a primrose or cowslip leaf you will see why these plants became associated with wrinkles. In 1551 William Tumer spoke out against the use of these plants:

'Some weomen, sprinkle ye floures of cowslip wt whyte wine and after still it and wash their faces wt that water to drive wrinkles away and to make them fayre in the eyes of the worlde rather than in the eyes of God, whom they are not afrayd to offend.'

GARLIC, that universal panacea, has also been used in the treatment of wrinkles, but those who dislike the smell will no doubt prefer to use ROSEMARY, which was said to have kept Elizabeth of Hungary wrinkle-free for many years. An old French lady told me that her youthful appearance was the result of washing with a mixture of 4g. ALUM and 200g. ROSEMARY infusion every night and morning and massaging this into the skin, working from chin to forehead.

Some wrinkle treatments utilise common garden vegetables. Raw POTATO or raw BEETROOT grated finely and mixed with a little whipped cream makes very good anti-wrinkle face masks.

A CREAM TO REMOVE WRINKLES
(from *Lotions and Potions*)

15g.   White wax
15g.   Spermaceti
30g.   Coconut oil
30g.   Lanolin
60g.   Sweet almond oil
3 drops Tincture of benzoin
         Orange-flower water

Melt the fats and oils in a porcelain dish. Remove from the fire, add orange-flower water and benzoin. Beat briskly until creamy. This should be massaged gently into the wrinkled area with the fingertips.

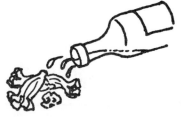

12 MOUTH, TEETH AND NOSE

Beautiful teeth are the work of nature, helped by a healthy diet, regular cleaning and a good dentist. Cleaning teeth nowadays automatically entails the use of toothpaste and the extensive toothpaste industry encourages us to go on thinking this way. A recent report from a consumers' organisation came to the conclusion that toothpastes do nothing to prevent tooth decay. They taste good and refresh the mouth. The fluoride in some pastes may help to prevent tooth decay in children but, even so, dentists prefer to prescribe fluoride in tablet form so that the dosage can be controlled.

Before toothpaste was invented herbal tooth powders were used to keep teeth clean. Dried SAGE was pounded into a fine powder and sprinkled on toothbrushes, or ROSEMARY twigs were burned to ashes and, before toothbrushes were invented, this was poured into linen bags which were used to polish the teeth: an old Flemish folk remedy claimed that this would 'kill the worms that make the holes in your teeth'. If worms in your teeth are not your problem try dissolving a little SEA SALT in water and cleaning your teeth with it. The taste is not as pleasant as toothpaste but it is just as efficient, and cheaper. Some herbalists recommend VERBENA infusion for cleaning the teeth, claiming that it helps resist decay.

Certainly, gargling with that fragrant liquid will counteract bad breath. LAVENDER tea can also be drunk or gargled to overcome halitosis; it also strengthens and disinfects the gums. BIRCH leaves and STRAWBERRY leaves in mouthwashes will help strengthen gums and sweeten the breath. ROSEMARY and WINE will also do this (see page 20). The white wine in the recipe is delicious but not essential.

W.M. suggests a more complicated recipe in *The Queen's Closet Opened*:

'Take the dried flowers and tops of rosemary, sugar candy, cloves, mace and cinnamon, of each a like quantity, dried and beaten into a fine powder, then take a new laid egg and pat the powder into the egg and sup off it fasting in the morning, do so seven days one after another and it will sweeten the breath.'

LEMON peel won't do much for your breath but if you rub it gently on your teeth and gums it will strengthen the latter and whiten the former.

The outside of your mouth may also present beauty problems of which the most common is probably dry, chapped lips. Some recipes to remedy this painful and unattractive complaint will be found later in this chapter. Two of the recipes contain SAGE which I have found to be most effective in the treatment of cold sores.

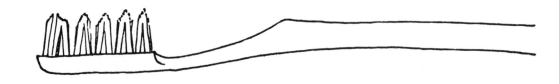

The problems most often associated with the nose are shininess and redness. Shininess is usually the result of localised over-oiliness of the skin. This can be treated with witch hazel infusion which will also help to reduce redness. Redness can also result from eating too much meat or heavily spiced food. If this is your problem it may be advisable to lay off the curry for a while. W.M. offers a delightful remedy for this imperfection:

For heat in the Face and Redness and Shinning of the nose

Take a fair linnen cloth, and in the morning lay it over the grass and draw it over till it is wet with dew, then wring it out into a fair dish and wet the face therewith as often as you please, as you wet it let it dry in. May dew is best.
    The Queen's Closet Opened, 1655

SPICY MOUTHWASH

20g.	Green aniseed
10g.	Star aniseed
5g.	Cloves
5g.	Cinnamon stick
10g.	Angelica
200g.	Alcohol 90°
3 drops	Mint oil

Steep the herbs and spices in the alcohol for about two weeks. Filter, and then add the mint oil. Add 1 teaspoon of this mixture to a glass of water and rinse the mouth. It will freshen the mouth and breath.

EXPENSIVE MOUTHWASH

30g.	Thyme
½ litre	Brandy

Steep the thyme in brandy for two weeks. Add 2 dessertspoons of the mixture to a glass of water. An extravagant but effective mouthwash.

To keepe the teeth both white and sound

Take a quart of honey as much vinegar and halfe so much white wine. Boyle them together and wash your teeth therewith now and then.
    Sir Hugh Platt, *Delights for Ladies*, 1609.

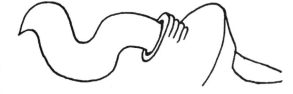

Definitely not recommended!

RED CLOVER SALVE

Fill a pan with red clover flowers. Cover these with
water. Bring to the boil and simmer for 1 hour.
Sieve, and press out all the liquid from the flowers.
Throw away the flowers and pour the water over a
panful of fresh clover heads. Repeat the process.
Reduce the liquid until it forms a thick syrup
(there will only be a small quantity). This Red
Clover Salve is an old folk remedy for dry and
splitting lips. It tastes very bitter but it is effective.

VIOLET SALVE

40g.   Essential oil of roses
15g.   Beeswax
40g.   Sweet violet infusion

Melt the wax and oil together, remove it from the
heat and beat in the violet infusion.

CHAPPED LIP OINTMENT

50g.   Beeswax
40g.   Spermaceti
40g.   Essential oil of sage

Melt the waxes gently then beat in the oil of sage.
Pour into a small pot or scoop it when cool into an
empty lipstick container. For chapped lips and
cold sores.

SAGE CREAM

40g.   Sweet almond oil
10g.   Beeswax
40g.   Rosewater
20g.   Dried sage

Melt the oil and wax together and add the sage.
Put this in the top of a double saucepan and leave
it to warm for 1—2 hours. Sieve and return it
briefly to a low heat. Gradually add the warmed
rosewater beating all the time. Remove from the
heat and continue beating until cool.

*An oil to take away the heat and shining of the
nose*

*Take six ounces of gourd seeds crack them, take
out the kernels and peel off the skins, blanch
three ounces of bitter almonds and make an oil
of them and anoint the nose with the oil, the
gourd seeds must weigh three ounces when
cracked.*
    Richard Pynsen, *A Proper New Booke of
    Cookerie*, 1576.

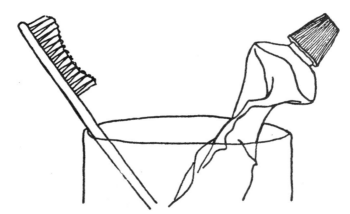

13 FRECKLES AND BLOTCHES

Freckles are fortunately no longer considered as ugly as they once were but then neither are they as fashionable as they were a few years ago when those not blessed with natural freckles adopted the extraordinary habit of painting small black spots on the nose. This practice, particularly popular in France, has now ceased.

Those who do want to get rid of freckles will of course have to stay out of the sun, but there are various herbs and simples which can help them.

Regular washing with an infusion of LIME flowers, PRIMROSE flowers or ROSEMARY are all said to bleach the skin. SCARLET PIMPERNEL infusion is another popular herbal 'anti-blotch and -freckle' herb. John Parkinson wrote in 1640 that French women 'account the distilled water of pimpernell mervailous good to cleanse the skin from any roughnesse deformity of discolouring thereof and to make it smooth neate and cleene'. He also gave a list of other plants: 'garden spurge, elder flowers, broom, madder, rue, gentian, scabious, betony, elecampane, Solomon's seal, the great hawkweed and lupin' are all recommended to 'cleanse the

skinne from freckles, sunburn and wrinkles'.

Better known as a bleaching agent is LEMON juice, but PARSLEY juice is also effective. Regular use of BUTTERMILK will also slowly help to bleach skin pigmentation and is more generally available than the 'hogsmilk' prescribed to remove freckles in an old Dutch herbal.

Squashed TOMATOES or EGGPLANT juice can be used to bleach freckles on the face when applied on a compress. CUCUMBER juice with the lemon juice added can be used in the same way or as a lotion.

Brown pigmentation of the skin resulting from over enthusiastic sunbathing or brownish coloured birth marks can also be bleached using these herbs and vegetables, or, perhaps most effectively, fresh HORSERADISH. Grate this finely and then pound it into a pulp, soften with a little lemon juice and bring it directly onto the skin or prepare the lotion described on page 38. *But do not use horseradish on your face. It stings and can cause irritation.*

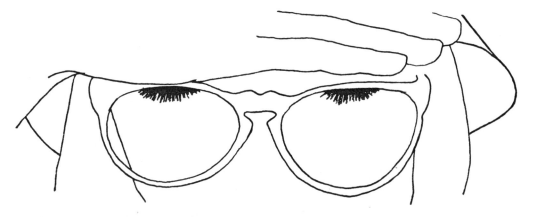

ANTI-FRECKLE CREAM: (a)

15g. White wax
15g. Spermaceti
100g. Essential oil of rosemary
50g. Lemon juice

Melt the spermaceti and white wax together. Gradually beat in warmed rosemary oil and lemon juice. Continue beating until cool.

ANTI-FRECKLE CREAM: (b)

1 Egg White
200g. Distilled water
10g. Icing sugar
The juice of 1 lemon

Beat the egg white until stiff and add the other ingredients gradually, beating all the time. Massage this mixture into your skin before sleeping. It is rather sticky but more effective than lemon juice alone.

ANTI-FRECKLE CREAM: (c)

½ litre Wine vinegar
1 Horseradish root finely grated

Put this mixture in a bottle. Seal it well and stand it in the sun for 2 days. Use this (but not on your face) before going to bed. The smell is rather strong but has the advantage of repelling mosquitos as well as bleaching the skin.

ANTI-FRECKLE CREAM: (d)

Pumpkin seed kernels
Olive oil

Pound the pumpkin seed kernels into a powder. Add just enough olive oil to form a paste. This is an ancient recipe. Keeps the skin soft and removes freckles.

To take away Spots and Freckles from the Face and Hands

The sap that issuith out of a birch tree in great abundance, being opened in March and April with a receiver of glass set under the boring thereof to catch the same, doth perform the same most excellently and maketh the skin very clear. This sap will dissolve pearls, a secret not known to many.

Sir Hugh Platt, *Delights for Ladies*, 1609

14 EYES

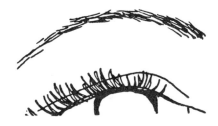 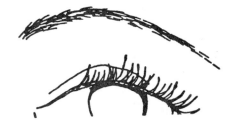

Eyelashes and eyebrows are, of course, hair. And very often, if you are giving your hair a herbal treatment, you can apply some to the eyebrows and lashes with a piece of cotton wool, making sure that it does not get into your eyes. But hair tonics containing alcohol must *never* be used near the eyes, whereas simple infusions, such as YARROW or ROSEMARY, are quite safe to use in this way.

Oil pomades are more conventional eyelash and eyebrow treatments. These are invaluable where the eyelashes have been damaged by excessive use of mascara, or where make-up has not been regularly and thoroughly removed before sleeping. Every night before going to bed rub a small amount of OLIVE OIL or ALMOND OIL into your eyelashes and they will become long, soft and silky. A mother of a friend of mine treated her daughter's lashes in this way from early childhood and the result was the longest and thickest eyelashes I have ever seen. But be careful, olive oil stings the eyes; use it with care.

Tired, irritated, red or swollen eyes can also respond to herbal eyebaths. A simple CAMOMILE infusion is particularly effective, but use distilled water and sieve very carefully through a muslin cloth. Swollen eyes may also be soothed by bathing them in a HORSETAIL decoction. FENNEL seed decoction is even better and the American Indians have even claimed that fennel seed eyebaths improve their sight.

For tired, dull eyes there is a simple and effective remedy. First rub a little cold cream round the eyes. Dip two pieces of cotton wool in WITCH HAZEL water. Lie down, close your eyes and lay the compresses on the eyelids. Relax for 10 minutes. The cold cream protects the sensitive skin round the eye from the astringency of the witch hazel.

Other eye compresses can be made by boiling a handful of CORNFLOWERS in ¼ litre distilled water. Simmer for 10 minutes. Cool, sieve, and use in the same way as the witch hazel. To remove 39

dark rings under the eyes use compressions of
LIME FLOWER tea in the same way as the other
compresses. Much more romantic is this seventeenth-century eye lotion:

'The morning dew that at a summer morning
forms on roses, will make the eyes clear and
pure.'

The same author also had a more practical
suggestion:

'To make tidy black eyebrows, burn a clove over a
candle, then dampen it with a little spit and draw
it over the eyebrows.'

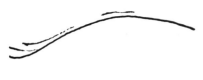

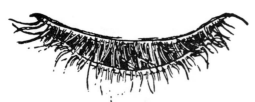

TO PREVENT THINNING EYEBROWS

10g.	Cornflower
10g.	Camomile
10g.	White dead-nettle
10g.	Sage leaves
10g.	Fumitory

Prepare a herbal infusion with 1 soupspoon
mixed herbs to 1 cup boiling water. Sieve. Use the
liquid warm to bathe the brows and lids.

EYELASH POMADE

1g.	Walnut juice
5g.	Castor oil
20g.	Vaseline
1 drop	Lavender oil (optional)

Melt the vaseline. Beat in the other ingredients.
Cool.

NOURISHING EYE CREAM

50g.	Essential oil of rosemary
25g.	Wheatgerm oil
25g.	Cocoa butter

Warm the ingredients gently together and beat
until cool. This cream is used to prevent
premature wrinkles around the eyes.

15 FACE MASKS AND COMPRESSES

Face masks provide a short but intensive treatment for the skin and never need to be applied more than once a week. Some people use them regularly but more often they are used to give the face an extra 'lift' for a special occasion, or after an illness when the complexion looks as run down as the body feels. The Spring is also a time for face masks, when the bright early sun shows up all the tiny flaws in your skin. A face mask will freshen you up as well as acting as a tonic for the skin. The greatest disadvantage of face masks is the time they take to prepare and apply. You have to be able to set aside at least 30 minutes to do nothing else. The mask has to be made, applied and left on for about 20 minutes. And it is very important that you relax completely while the pack is on, if the full benefit of it is to be achieved.

There are face masks for every possible skin type and it can be great fun to experiment with the various substances used. Virtually every fruit and vegetable has been used in a face mask at some time or other. The juice is usually mixed with FULLER'S EARTH or simply pulped and spread over the face. Herbal infusions (chosen to suit your skin type as described in Chapter 4) can also be mixed with fuller's earth to make 'mud' packs which are just as beneficial for human beings as for hippopotamuses.

One excellent nourishing face mask which will cleanse, nourish and tone up the complexion and which is suitable for most skin types is made with EGG YOLK and LEMON. Take ½ lemon and hollow out just enough of the inside to hold 1 egg yolk. Put the unbroken yolk into the lemon and leave it overnight. As always before applying a mask cleanse your face and neck thoroughly and then dry it slowly. Cover your face and neck with a warm towel for a minute or two to open the pores. Spread the mixture, in this case the egg yolk which will have absorbed some of the citrus oils, evenly over the face avoiding the area round the eyes. Relax for about 20 minutes. Wash the mask off with lukewarm water. This process can be

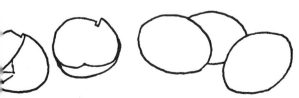

followed for all face masks. For an 'instant' version of the above mask simply beat an egg yolk with 1 teaspoon ORANGE, lemon, or CUCUMBER juice, but this is not as effective as the original one. Another nourishing and soothing mask can be prepared by beating 1 egg yolk with a walnut of fresh YEAST, and a few drops of SWEET ALMOND OIL. A very dry flaky skin will benefit even more from an egg yolk beaten with 1 teaspoon OLIVE OIL — a simple but unbeatable remedy. This mask can be removed with lukewarm MILK if the skin is very sensitive.

EGG WHITES are only used in astringent face masks. For a very oily skin, beat an egg white stiffly and add a few drops of herbal infusion or lemon juice to improve the skin tone. A more nourishing mixture can be made with beaten egg white and a teaspoon of HONEY.

Fruit masks are also lightly astringent and will improve the tone and texture of the skin. Purees of STRAWBERRIES, PEACHES or APRICOTS are some of the most popular. These can be mixed with WHIPPED CREAM for a dry skin, or egg yolk for an oily one. There is, however, no evidence that vitamins are absorbed through the skin as commercial cosmetic companies so often claim.

The two most often used vegetable cosmetics are CUCUMBER and AVOCADO. Cucumbers are refreshing, soothing and slightly astringent. Avocados are emollient and nourishing but expensive. Raw purées of these can be used by themselves or mixed with one of the cereals described later.

SPINACH boiled gently in milk can be used to good effect on a flaky skin. Raw POTATOES or BEETROOT grated and mixed with a little cream are said to work wonders for wrinkles. Strawberries are also supposed to help smoothe out tiny lines and wrinkles.

Various cereals form the basis of cleansing and nourishing face masks. CORNFLOUR, BARLEY MEAL and OATMEAL can all be mixed to a paste with distilled water or herbal infusions. GROUND ALMONDS can be used in the same way and this leaves the skin feeling wonderfully soft and silky.

Whereas face masks are thick and pasty enough to be applied directly to the face compresses may be made with pieces of absorbent linen for applying liquids which are too runny to be used in this way. Cut a square of linen somewhat larger than your face and cut holes for the eyes and mouth. Dip this into your liquid and lay it over your face. Leave it on for about 20 minutes and then rinse your face thoroughly with soft water. YOGHURT, BUTTERMILK, milk, herbal infusions and fruit juices can all be applied in this way. The compresses will act as a moisturiser and cleanser but they do not tone up the face as effectively as do masks. On the other hand they are gentle and much more suitable for delicate skin. A compress which herbalists recommend very highly is one made with an infusion of ST. JOHN'S WORT. This is a natural moisturiser and should be used if your skin is feeling rather dry and tight. Rinse your face after using it with a little buttermilk, if available.

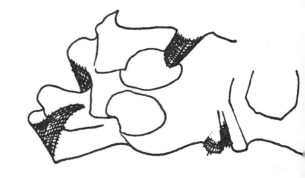

16 BODY PACKS

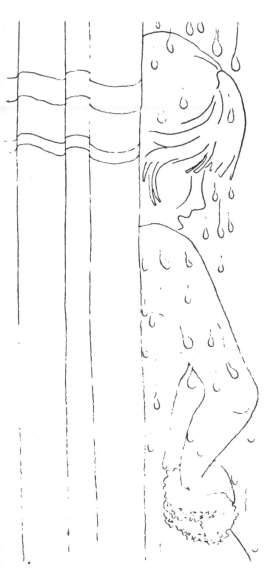

A body pack is obviously not something that most people will want to apply very often. Only the courtesan with nothing to do but wait for her lover can ever have enough time to go in for body packs in a big way. Time, energy, and preferably someone to clean the bath afterwards, are all needed. However there are some occasions when you will want to look your best all over. They can tone up your skin after the winter and improve your first appearance in beach outfits.

OATMEAL is one of the messiest but most effective body packs. It removes impurities from the skin and improves tone and texture. Mix the oatmeal into a fine paste with water, or even better, buttermilk, and smear it over the clean warm dry body. Find something washable to sit on and leave the pack on for about 15 minutes. Wash off with lukewarm water. (See also below for an easier if less thorough way of cleansing with oatmeal.)

LEMON juice makes an astringent body pack which will also improve skin colour. Mix the juice with oatmeal or prepare a decoction of washed, sliced whole lemons and ORANGES (including the skins). Slice 2 lemons and 2 oranges, or 4 lemons, and simmer these in 2 litres water for ½ hour. Cool, sieve, and sponge the mixture slowly and gently all over your body.

A MILK bath, so beneficial to Cleopatra, is rather expensive even when cow's milk rather than the, for most of us unobtainable, ass's milk is used. But 1 litre milk mixed with the juice of 2 lemons, sponged over the body and left on for 10–15 minutes is a good substitute. It is certainly more effective than the usual modern version, which is to empty a packet of dried milk into the bath water.

For a really sticky mess try beating 4 eggs with the juice of 4 lemons and smear yourself with this. It is said to be good for oily, spotty skin and it will certainly have an astringent and purifying action. Less sticky are YOGHURT and BUTTERMILK which can also be sponged over the body. These will have a mild bleaching, softening and cleansing effect.

43

17 BEAUTY BATHS

Taking baths was for many centuries considered to be a dangerous and unpleasant chore. It was rarely done to cleanse the body but herbal baths were sometimes used as cures. It is thought to have been a herbal bath that Marat was sitting in when he was murdered by Charlotte Corday. He suffered from an unpleasant but undefined skin disease. The use of herbal baths in medicine has now virtually died out but there is renewed interest in cosmetic herbal baths which are certainly cheaper and pleasanter than the Countess of Bathory's blood of murdered virgins. Alcohol also seems to have gone out of fashion: film stars no longer bath in champagne and I have never heard of anyone prepared to follow the example of Mary Queen of Scots who regularly wallowed in red wine.

Herbal baths can be refreshing, stimulating, fragrant and even sleep-inducing. Usually a strong decoction or infusion is added to the bath water but there are some who find it more romantic to add a few fresh flowers or leaves and bath surrounded by greenery which later has to be cleared up.

ROSEMARY and LAVENDER are perhaps the two most popular bathing herbs. A strong decoction of either of these will impart a delicious perfume to the bath water. In summer a sprig of either will be just as effective and not too messy. As well as perfuming the bath lavender is a disinfectant and will soften your skin. Its perfume is also said to strengthen the nerves. Rosemary will stimulate the circulation and glandular action. PEPPERMINT infusion is an invigorating addition to the water, while CAMOMILE will soothe the nerves and soften the skin. For a truly relaxing and sleep-inducing bath add a little VALERIAN decoction. The perfume isn't so pleasant but it will improve your night's rest, and is said to be very beneficial for nervous children who suffer from nightmares.

Even commercial deodorants are replaceable. OAKLEAF infusion is an excellent deodorant, and LOVAGE also makes a refreshing bath that keeps you fragrant. HORSETAIL, that interesting garden weed, can be made into a decoction which can be added to the bath to heal small scratches and abrasions: just the thing if you have been walking through a bramble patch.

ROSE petals or HONEYSUCKLE leaves and flowers will keep your skin soft as well as perfuming the water. Ovid recommended LUPIN flowers for a scintillating tonic bath. To really soften rough or chapped skin add a few drops of ALMOND OIL. Or prepare an essential oil using almond oil and your choice of herb to get the best of both worlds. Lavender oil is the most popular.

MIXED HERBAL BATH

10g.	Rosemary
10g.	Thyme
10g.	Lavender
10g.	Marjoram
10g.	Sage

Prepare a decoction of these herbs using 3 dessertspoons herbal mixture to 1 litre water. Sieve and bottle. Add 1 cup of this to your bath water. You can add brandy to preserve it if you feel extravagant but it should keep in the refrigerator for 2—3 weeks without it.

PINE BATH EXTRACT

Boil clean young pine needles and cones with five times their volume of water. Simmer for 40 minutes then press out all the liquid into a saucepan. Reduce this by boiling, until it thickens. Add 150g. extract to one bath. This makes a very stimulating bath which invigorates the circulation. Do not use more than the recommended dose as this closes the pores.

SEVENTEENTH-CENTURY AROMATIC BATH

Bay leaves
Thyme
Rosemary
Marjoram
Lavender
Wormwood
Pennyroyal (or another mint)
Lemon balm
Peppermint
Brandy

Take a handful of each of these fresh herbs (1 dessertspoon dried) and boil them for 10 minutes in 2 litres water. Sieve the mixture and add ½ bottle brandy. Pour a little of this into your bath. This recipe comes from *The Toilet of Flora* a seventeenth-century manual. It is well worth trying, and poured into pretty bottles it makes a very acceptable present. The brandy acts as a preservative.

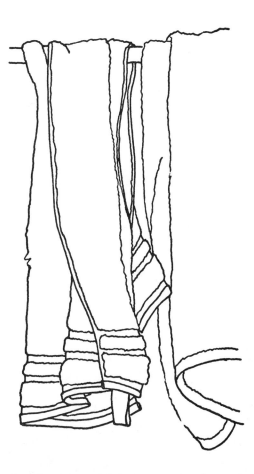

45

HERBAL BATH OIL

5g.   Essential oil of thyme
2g.   Essential oil of marjoram
2g.   Essential oil of lavender
1 glass Brandy

Shake the oils together in the brandy and add a
teaspoonful of this mixture to your bath. It is less
greasy than using the oils alone.

LAVENDER BATH EXTRACT

3 handfuls Fresh lavender flowers
½ litre   Brandy
30g.   Orange blossom water
30g.   Rosewater
60g.   Distilled water
5g.   Essential oil of lavender

Pour the brandy over the fresh lavender flowers
and leave it to stand for 3 days. Sieve carefully.
Add the lavender oil, orange blossom water, rosewater and distilled water. Shake well and keep in
an airtight bottle.

OATMEAL BATH

Sew some little bags of cheesecloth and fill these
with oatmeal. Rub your entire body with these in
the bath. The bags can be used more than once
and they will remove many of the impurities from
your skin.

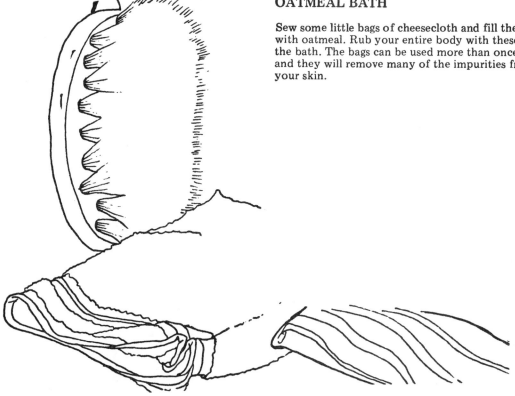

18 HAIR LOTIONS

Hair lotions are strong solutions which will improve hair condition and stimulate growth. Unfortunately they are not hair restorers. Balding in men is usually hormonal and there is nothing that these potions can do to make hair grow on a bald head. But it isn't for lack of trying. Hair restorers have been an important part of every herbal and household manual since the Ancient Greeks and no doubt before that. Ancient books are filled with extraordinary mixtures, all intended to make hair grow. Some of these seem more likely to scalp the unfortunate victims but herbalists seldom mention their failures. Important ingredients of these potions included bear grease, ashes of bees, and mouse or goat's dung. It would be possible, if not constructive, to fill an entire chapter with these fascinating mixtures.

Most of the hair lotions mentioned here are simple solutions of various ingredients in alcohol. In most cases they have to stand for several days and then be filtered. A coffee filter is ideal for this purpose but some lotions will still have to be filtered several times until the liquid is completely clear.

Hair lotions containing alcohol do not need to be used more than once or twice a week. Overdoses could cause the scalp to become dry and flaky. The lotions should be rubbed gently into the head with a piece of cotton wool or a soft brush. It will be more effective if you follow this up by massaging the scalp with the finger tips. Never use too much liquid or it can run down into your eyes, which is both painful and dangerous.

The ingredients for all these lotions simply need shaking together. But when the lotion has been left to stand the oily ingredients will float to the top. The lotions will always need to be shaken before use. The tinctures used in the lotions can be bought at some homoeopathic chemists, or they can be made as described in Chapter 3.

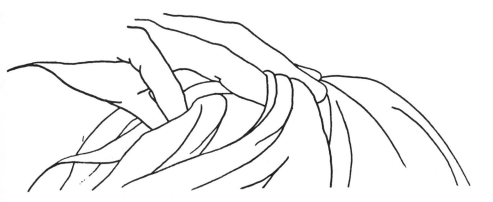

TO PREVENT SEBORRHOEA AND FALLING HAIR

a.
20g.   Rum
25g.   Castor oil
25g.   Peruvian bark or chillies
100g. Alcohol
100g. Eau de Cologne

Steep the Peruvian bark or chillies in alcohol for 3 days. Sieve. Add to the other ingredients. Massage this into the scalp twice a week.

b.
60g.   Alcohol
5g.   Tincture of Peruvian bark or chillies
1g.   Peruvian balsam
5g.   Orange blossom water
3g.   Rosemary tincture

A stimulating aromatic mixture.

c.
60g.   Alcohol
10g.   Arnica tincture
1 drop Peruvian balsam
30g.   Distilled water
2 drops Rosemary oil

A softer mixture for a more delicate skin. Also very aromatic.

CAMOMILE LOTION FOR BLOND HAIR

50g.   Alcohol
20g.   Camomile tincture
10g.   St John's wort tincture
30g.   Rosewater

LOTIONS WITH FRESH NETTLES

Nettles are very good for your hair. They stimulate the circulation of the scalp and improve hair condition.

a.
Take one part of fresh stinging nettles to three parts alcohol. Let the mixture stand for two weeks in the sun. Filter carefully. Use 3 teaspoons of this tincture to 250g. water. Massage daily into the scalp.

b.
100g. Fresh stinging nettles
500g. Water
500g. White wine vinegar

Simmer the chopped young nettles in water and white wine vinegar for ½ hour. Sieve well. Massage a little into the scalp daily. Unfortunately this excellent lotion has a rather unattractive smell.

LOTION WITH NETTLE TINCTURE

50g.   Alcohol
30g.   Nettle tincture
1 drop   Peruvian balsam
30g.   Orange blossom water
A few drops Lavender oil

This is a more complicated but more refined formula than the two preceding recipes and certainly more fragrant than the nettle/vinegar mixture. The simpler recipes containing fresh nettles are, however, equally effective. Use this lotion 2 or 3 times a week.

ANTISEPTIC HAIR LOTION WITH GARLIC

55g.   Alcohol
5g.   Garlic extract or 1 crushed bulb of fresh garlic
40g.   Distilled water

Garlic will stimulate hair growth and help prevent dandruff. Smell is the problem. If you are using fresh garlic let it steep in the alcohol for 3 days. Filter and add the water. Perfume to taste.

ANTISEPTIC HAIR LOTION WITH BIRCH TINCTURE

53g.   Alcohol
10g.   Birch leaf tincture
10g.   Birch bud tincture
25g.   Water

An excellent lotion to condition the hair and to stimulate hair growth. Rosemary or lavender oil can be added to perfume it.

To make hair grow thick

Take a good quantity of the roots of hyssop, burn them to ashes, make a strong lye, mingle them with ashes and wash the head with it. The ashes of goats dung mixed with oil will have the same effect.
    The Queen's Closet Opened, 1655

An ointment to cause the hair to grow

Take a quarter of a pound of bears grease, put to this two drams of the ashes of southernwood, two drams of the ashes of burnt bees, two drams of sweet almonds and two drams of the juice of white lilly root and eight drams of musk. Make an ointment of these. Shave the place where the hair is wanted the day before the full of the moon and it will cause it to grow.
    The Queen's Closet Opened, 1655

In case that a man be bald, Plinius the mickle leech saith this leechdom:

Take dead bees, burn them to ashes, add oil upon that, seethe very long over gledes, then strain, wring out and take leaves of willow, pound them, pour the juice into the oil, boil again for a while on gledes, strain them, smear therewith after the bath.
    The Leech Book of Bald

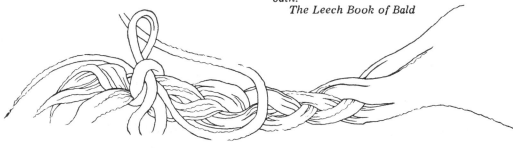

19 HAIR RINSES

These rinses are mostly simple herbal infusions or decoctions. They cannot be kept for longer than a few days, but they are so simple to make that it is worth brewing a pot of fresh 'herb tea' to rinse your hair after every wash. The rinses are not as strong as the hair tonics in the previous chapter and are used more as a preventative to keep the hair in good condition than as a cure. Regular use of them really does help to keep hair in the peak of condition.

LIME FLOWER infusion is one old and tried way to keep your hair soft and shining. An infusion of BIRCH LEAVES or, even stronger, a decoction of BIRCH BUDS will have the same effect. BIRCH SAP is also excellent for conditioning hair. It can be collected in early Spring by making a deep cut in the tree trunk when the sap will run out slowly and can be caught in a bowl. A spoonful of this in the last rinse water will act as a splendid Spring cure for your hair.

ROSEMARY decoction makes a fragrant and effective rinse for people with dark hair. Simmer a small bunch of fresh rosemary (or 2 dessertspoons dried) for ½ hour in ½ litre water. CAMOMILE infusion is more suitable for blond hair.

John Parkinson claimed in 1629 that 'the ashes of southernwood mixed with old salad oil will cause a beard to grow, or hair on a bald head'. He also recommended YARROW and indeed both these herbs, if not quite the miracle-workers he described, will improve hair condition. Yarrow will also help to clear up mild cases of dandruff. More acute dandruff can be treated with infusions of BURDOCK, HORSETAIL or COLTSFOOT. However it must be emphasised that persistent dandruff, particularly if it is accompanied by a sore or irritated scalp *must* be diagnosed by a doctor. It may turn out to be something else altogether.

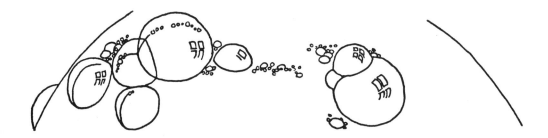

ARNICA can help prevent dandruff and stimulate the circulation in the scalp. Like PERUVIAN BARK it is used in many commercial hair preparations and can be obtained from herbalists. PERUVIAN BARK is one of the most effective cures for seborrhoea. It is also said to stimulate hair growth and prevent hair loss. The same is said for CHILLIES which is also an ingredient in many hair lotions.

Infusions of ROSE, JASMINE, VIOLET and LAVENDER will impart a lasting fragrance to your hair which makes the use of commercial perfumes completely unnecessary.

BEER has a less attractive smell but it remains the simplest way of giving body to your hair, and is a much better setting lotion than the sticky mixtures many people use. But make sure you use a good quality natural beer: many beers sold nowadays are chemically produced and contain various synthetic ingredients.

MAIDENHAIR FERN conjures up a picture of antimacassars, grand pianos and formal floral arrangements but they are not merely decorative. Maidenhair infusions will prevent hair loss and stimulate its growth. CLEAVERS, whose silky strands provide so much amusement for country children, makes one of nature's best hair tonics. Infuse a handful of chopped cleavers in ½ litre boiling water. Finally, a really prosaic cure for oily seborrhoea: SAUERKRAUT juice should be rubbed into the scalp with a piece of cotton wool daily until the condition improves. It is neither fragrant nor in any way attractive but it does work. This juice can be bought ready prepared at health food shops.

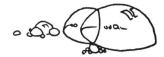

20 HAIR COLOURANTS

There are as many natural ways of tinting your hair, as there are commercial preparations. Natural methods often work more slowly but will frequently act as hair conditioners as well as colourants. Chemical hair dyes often contain irritant substances which can cause allergies and damage hair and scalp. Indeed many of these commercial preparations and shampoos to colour the hair are sold as 'herbal' but the quantities of herbs are never mentioned and it is doubtful if many of their qualities are preserved after they have been steeped in detergents.

It is so little bother to prepare a herbal infusion it must be worthwhile to prepare your own rinses so that you know exactly what goes into them.

CAMOMILE is certainly the best known herb for blond and light brown hair. It has a mild bleaching action and will impart a rich golden sheen to the hair. Dried or fresh herbs are equally effective in this case and it is such a common weed that it is simple to pick enough CAMOMILE in one afternoon to last the entire winter. Use 2 dessertspoonfuls of dried herbs to ½ litre of water.

LEMON is also an excellent bleach and will improve the condition of greasy hair without the use of strong detergents. Add the juice of one lemon to ½ litre of water and rinse your hair with this after every wash. It will keep your hair light after it has been bleached by the summer sun, but it must be used regularly. QUINCE juice added to the last rinsewater will also give a golden shine to light hair.

John Parkinson wrote 'The Golden flowers of Mullein boiled in lye dyeth the hairs of the head yellow and maketh them fair and smooth' but I can't imagine lye doing anyone's hair much good.

William Tumer (1551) disapproved of hair dyes, of MARIGOLD he commented 'Summe use to make theyr here yellow with the floure of this herbe, not being content with the naturall colour which God hath given them.'

Ordinary household TEA can also be used as a hair colourant. Light-midbrown hair will acquire an attractive chestnut shine if pots of tea are poured over it regularly.

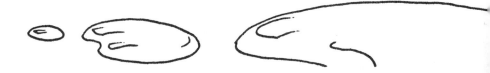

It is said that Titian's models used PRIVET leaves to give their hair that particular copper glow. But as every hippy knows it is EGYPTIAN PRIVET or HENNA which can really dye your hair semi-permanently red. Many would-be users are rather put off by the bright orange colour which henna dyes very blond or bleached hair. But on dark or middle brown hair it can give beautiful coppery colours, and above all it is a fantastic hair conditioner. Some even claim that it causes the individual hairs to swell and therefore thickens the hair. What is certain is that a henna treatment will leave the hair supple, shining and easy to handle. Before using henna test a little on one strand of hair. Those with lighter coloured hair will find they don't want to leave it on for more than 10—15 minutes to get the desired chestnut gleam. On the other hand those with dark hair may want to leave it on overnight to get the maximum colouring and conditioning effect.

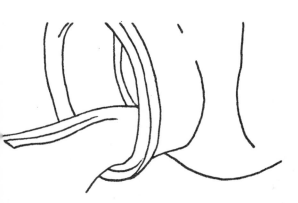

Henna is bought in powder form. Mix this into a thick paste with boiling water. Add a few drops of vinegar or lemon juice and leave to cool. Wash your hair thoroughly and smear a little cold cream around the hair line to prevent the skin becoming stained. Using plastic gloves to protect your hands apply the warm henna paste to the clean damp hair. Be careful to apply it evenly all over the head. It is easiest to divide your hair into sections with a comb and deal with one section at a time. You will then ensure that the henna gets to the hair roots. Use a shower cap to cover the head and leave on as long as necessary. It is also possible to buy NEUTRAL HENNA to use as a conditioner and BLACK HENNA (mixed with indigo) to darken the hair. Henna has been used all over the east, at least since the time of the Ancient Egyptians.

More recently, 100—200 years ago, TOBACCO was a widely used hair dye, to disguise grey hairs. Used regularly on brown—dark brown hair it can be effective. Prepare a decoction using 1 dessert-spoon dark tobacco to ½ litre water. Light brown hair going grey can be rinsed with an infusion of tea and tobacco: 1 teaspoonful of each to ½ litre water. According to Simon Witgeest (1715) daily washes with GOAT'S MILK was a remedy for grey hair 'proven a thousand times'!

To darken the hair or intensify the colour of dark hair try an infusion of ROSEMARY and RED SAGE. It smells deliciously spicy and is a good conditioner but it has to be used regularly to have a darkening effect. The Romans used a decoction of ELDERBERRIES to give their dark hair an intensified colour and shine.

FOR BLACK HAIR

100g. The outer green covering of walnuts
500g. Alcohol
A few drops of essential oil of rosemary

Steep the walnut skins in the alcohol for 10 days.
Sieve. Perfume with rosemary oil. Rub a small
quantity of this into the hair after washing.

FOR BLOND HAIR

100g. Rhubarb
20g. Camomile flowers
1 litre Water
5g. Borax (optional)

Boil the rhubarb and camomile in water until the
liquid is reduced by half. Cool and add the borax
which acts as an emulsifying agent. Add a cupful
of this to ½ litre water and rinse the hair with it.

AGAINST GREY HAIR

1 dessertspoon Tea
1 dessertspoon Dried sage
1 dessertspoon Rum
1 litre Water

Simmer the tea and sage in water for 2 hours. Cool
and sieve. Add the rum. Rub this mixture into the
hair four or five times a week.

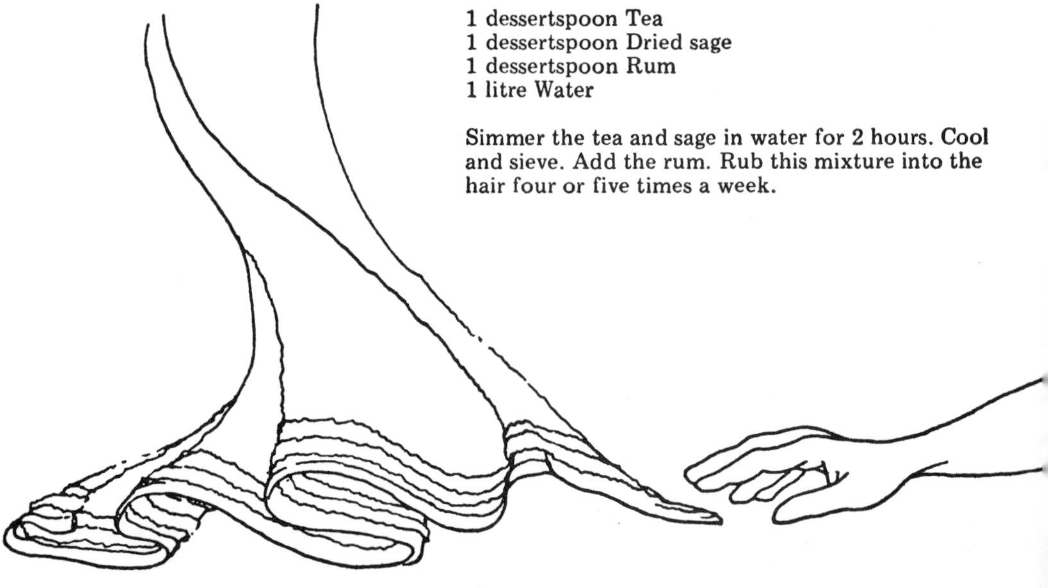

SHAMPOO FOR BLOND HAIR

2 dessertspoons Dried camomile flowers
The juice of ½ lemon
150g. Castile soap
1 litre Water

Prepare an infusion of the camomile flowers and water. Let it cool. Add the lemon juice. Grate the soap and dissolve it in the infusion. Bring it gently to the boil stirring occasionally until the water is clear. Remove from the heat and beat until the mixture is fluffy.

SHAMPOO FOR DARK HAIR

Prepare in the same way as the previous recipe but substitute red sage or rosemary for the camomile flowers and leave out the lemon juice.

How to colour the head or beard into a chestnut colour in half an houre: (if you survive the treatment!)

Take one part of lead caleined with sulphur and one parte of quicke lime, temper them somewhat with water, let it upon the haire chafing it well in and let it dry one quarter of an houre or there-abouts. Then wash the same off with faire water divers times and lastly with soape and water and it will be a verie naturall haire colour. The longer it lyeth upon the hair the browner it groweth. This coloures not the flesh at all and yet it lasteth very long in the haire.
W.M., *The Queen's Closet Opened,* 1655

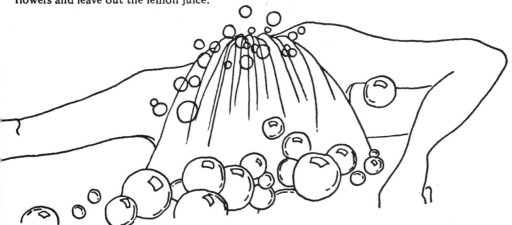

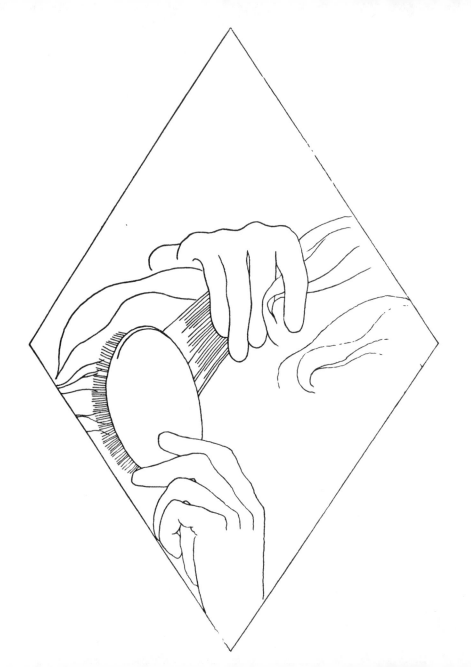

21 TIPS TO IMPROVE HAIR CONDITION

Apart from the herbal rinses and tonics there are many natural ways of keeping the hair well conditioned. Some are simple, others more complicated. Hair massages are a simple way to improve the hair condition. Take a good quality bristle brush and standing by an open window brush your hair very thoroughly from the back of the head to the forehead. This will stimulate the circulation in your scalp and 'air' your hair. A tense scalp can also have a detrimental effect on your hair. This can be relieved by a dry massage. Place your hands on your head and massage the scalp with your palms, or better still find someone else to do it for you.

If you have time before washing your hair to give your scalp a wet massage you will stimulate the growth of your hair. Wet your hair and beginning at the nape of your head knead your scalp with the finger tips, keeping the fingers well spread. Repeat this process beginning from the temples and forehead and working to the back of the head.

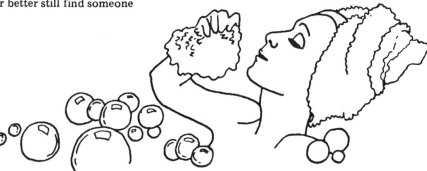

Dry hair can be greatly improved by massaging in this way with ALMOND OIL. After massaging the oil into the head wrap a warm towel around your hair to increase the absorption. Wash your hair thoroughly after 20 minutes. The same treatment will successfully clear up dandruff. It also has the advantage that it soothes rather than irritates the skin as some strong antiseptic products do. It is therefore very suitable for sensitive skins.

OLIVE OIL is another feeding anti-dandruff treatment which is used for fine, easily damaged, and difficult to manage hair. It is best to give your hair an intensive treatment with olive oil so that as much of it as possible is absorbed. Apply it in the same way as the almond oil but try to leave it on for at least 6 hours, or overnight. You will of course need to cover your head with a plastic hat and protect the pillow with an old towel. Wash out the oil thoroughly next morning. Your hair will be left shining and manageable. This treatment makes an excellent cure for the hair after the summer holidays, when it is often dry and brittle from the sun and sea.

Try rubbing your scalp with a clove of GARLIC. It sounds like an old wives' tale but it isn't. Garlic is very good for the hair and a well known treatment to prevent hair loss and increase blood circulation in the scalp. It is a strong antiseptic and is a useful anti-seborrhoea treatment. The smell may put you off but a good herbal shampoo (opposite) will wash away the smell. A more refined garlic treatment can be found in Chapter 18. ONION can be used in the same way as garlic but is considerably milder. You can also rinse your hair with onion decoction. The smell is then still present but is less penetrating.

EGG YOLK is not as odorous and is a better-known hair conditioner. There are of course hundreds of egg shampoos to be found in the shops but often the amount of egg contained is minimal. A 'do-it-yourself' egg treatment is much more effective.

Take one lightly beaten egg yolk and rub this into your damp hair. Leave it on for 10 minutes and then rinse with lukewarm water. Make sure this is not too hot or you will end up with scrambled egg in your hair, which is very difficult to wash out.

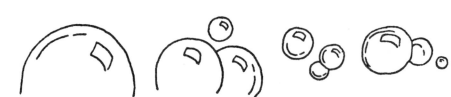

The condition of very oily hair can be improved by adding 1 teaspoon natural SEA SALT to every 50 grams of shampoo. Do not wash your hair with very hot water and do not be alarmed if the lather is reduced. Your hair will still be clean.

The addition of LEMON juice to the last rinse water will also help to keep the hair less oily and will impart a sheen to it. But it will bleach the hair slightly.

VINEGAR will also give your hair that extra shine. Add 1 dessertspoonful to your last rinse water.

CIDER VINEGAR will clear up dandruff and can be massaged into the scalp 3 or 4 times a week. This is a most effective treatment but leaves your hair smelling of apple vinegar, not an unpleasant odour but hardly a delicate perfume. Culpeper also recommends WILD MINT infused in vinegar as 'an excellent wash to get rid of scurf'.

HERBAL SHAMPOOS

a.
Sage
Rosemary
Thyme
Yarrow
Nettles
Distilled Water
Castile soap

Prepare an infusion using 2—3 dessertspoons each fresh herb (or 1 dessertspoon dried herb) to 1 litre distilled water. Sieve and add 150g. grated castile soap and bring the mixture slowly to the boil, stirring all the time until the water is clear. Remove from the heat and beat the mixture until it is fluffy. Pour into a jar.

b.
1 handful Birch buds and leaves
1 teaspoon Fresh birch juice
1 handful Fresh nettles
1 litre Water
150g. Grated castile soap

Prepare as in the preceding recipe.

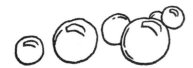

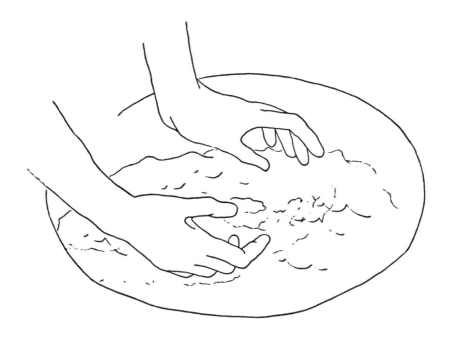

22 HANDS

One might think that hands would need less attention nowadays than in the bad old days of really heavy housework, when floors and tables had to be scrubbed and grates blackened. This is not so. Detergents dry out the skin and cause as much damage to the hands as the rubbing and scrubbing used to do. Rubber gloves are one answer to this but many people find these uncomfortable to wear. It is more practical to change from detergents to the cleaning products based on Panama wood, which do not play havoc with your hands and do not pollute the environment in the way that detergents do.

But hands get damaged in many other ways. Gardening, cooking and painting are all pleasurable pastimes but they can leave you with discoloured, rough hands, and there are still many people whose everyday work makes the use of hand-creams essential.

A simple way to prevent chapped hands and to keep them soft is to add a teaspoonful of OLIVE or ALMOND OIL to the water in your hand basin when you wash your hands. If you keep a small bottle of oil on the hand basin and use it regularly this is a very effective treatment, although it inevitably leaves the hand basin unpleasantly greasy.

Herbs will also help to keep hands soft and white. CAMOMILE infusion makes a good herbal hand lotion. In 1732 Charles Carter mentioned another herb 'To Take staines out of ones hands presently. This is done with the juyce of SORREL washing the stained place therein'.

GROUNDSEL is not only for the birds. It has long been used for its healing qualities and a hand bath in groundsel infusion will quicken the healing of small cuts, abrasions and chapped skin. After the hand bath dry your hands thoroughly and apply one of the hand creams given at the end of this chapter. OAK BARK decoction has a similar healing action.

Red hands, often the result of poor circulation, can be prevented by baths in HAZEL leaf and EUCALYPTUS leaf decoction. Boil a handful of each of these leaves in a litre of water for about ½ hour. Sieve this and bathe your hands in the hot decoction for 10 minutes. Dry your hands and rub a little OATMEAL into them.

GLYCERINE forms the basis of most hand creams but if you don't have time to make these you can massage a little pure glycerine mixed with a few drops of essential oil of LAVENDER into your hands. Less sticky is a mixture of equal quantities of glycerine and LEMON juice which will keep hands soft and white. These lotions should be used nightly.

Hands which are already badly chapped or roughened can be improved by baths in warm ALMOND OIL. This is rather expensive but it can be kept specially for this purpose and used again and again. It is particularly good for people whose hands are constantly exposed to water and cold. After bathing the hands in almond oil wash them in warm soft water using a mild unperfumed soap and apply glycerine hand cream.

Sufferers from chilblains can gain relief by massaging beaten EGG WHITE or whipped CREAM into their hands, or by hand baths in HAZEL leaf infusion. Other chilblain remedies can be found in Chapter 23 and in the recipes which follow.

These recipes can also be used as a vehicle for your favourite herbs. Use one of the herbs just mentioned, or LAVENDER for its antiseptic qualities and perfume, or ELDER flowers which soften and whiten the hands. Remember that, as before, the asterisk indicates where a simple substance can be replaced by a herbal preparation.

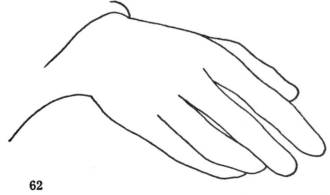

GLYCERINE JELLY

3 dessertspoons	Glycerine
6 dessertspoons	Rosewater *
2 teaspoons	Eau de Cologne
2 teaspoons	Gum tragacanth

Dissolve the gum in the eau de Cologne. Shake the rosewater or herbal infusion with the glycerine and beat this into the gum and eau de Cologne mixture.

LANOLIN HAND CREAM

100g.	Lanolin
100g.	White vaseline
10g.	Almond oil *
10g.	Rosewater

Warm the vaseline and lanolin together and gradually beat in the essential oil or almond oil and rosewater. Take this mixture from the heat and continue beating for 10 minutes with an electric mixer. Leave it overnight and beat it again the following morning.

LEMON LOTION

Rosewater *
Lemon juice
Glycerine
Alcohol 50°

Mix equal quantities of these ingredients in a bottle and shake well.

POTATO CREAM

Boil a few good 'floury' potatoes. Mash them well and add enough milk and rosewater in equal quantity to make the potato into a thick cream. Add a few drops of glycerine. Massage this daily into your hands to keep them soft and white. It will keep for about a week in the refrigerator.

ELDERFLOWER HAND LOTION

Shake together 5 parts glycerine to 15 parts elder-flower infusion.

WINTER HAND LOTION

5g.   Peruvian balsam
13g.   Benzoin tincture
125g. Alcohol 90°

Shake the ingredients well together. Rub it into your hands morning and evening during cold weather and it will help to prevent chilblains and chapped hands.

FINGERNAILS

The worst beauty problem with fingernails must be the urge that some people have to bite them. A recent psychiatric report says that it has nothing to do with having a neurotic personality. In fact, the causes of nailbiting remain a mystery. Nor has anyone yet found an effective cure. People used to put BITTER ALOES on their children's nails to discourage the habit, but it doesn't always work.

Even people who do not bite their nails can have problems with brittle, easily broken nails. This can be partially remedied by oil baths. Dabble your fingers in warm ALMOND OIL. If they are in very bad condition do this every evening for 8 minutes. Then take a cotton wool tipped stick and very gently push back the cuticles. OLIVE OIL can also be used in this way. If you add a few drops of LEMON juice to the oil bath it will help strengthen your nails. Alternatively rub the nails with lemon juice in the mornings and bathe them in oil in the evenings.

HORSETAIL is the most effective herbal remedy for poor fingernails. Bathe the nails in horsetail decoction or take it internally. Jean Palaiseul in *Grandmother's Secrets* suggests '40—50 grams of dried plant (horsetail) gathered in July—August, to a litre of water; cold soak for a minimum of three hours, heat and simmer gently for twenty to twenty-five minutes. Leave to infuse for ten minutes, 3—4 cupfuls per day. This decoction taken regularly for two to three weeks will cause white spots on the fingernails to disappear ... breaking nails, a sign of decalcification, become normal again in a fortnight if horsetail extract is taken, and in a slightly longer time if the less concentrated decoction is taken'. According to Palaiseul the effectiveness of horsetail is due to its very high mineral content.

If the nails are weak and brittle it is advisable not to use nail polish and acetone on them as this will make them even weaker. Polish them instead with a little GLYCERINE. To encourage nail growth, dissolve 2 teaspoons GELATINE in a glass of ORANGE juice and drink this every morning.

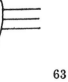

23 LEGS AND FEET

Beautiful shapely legs are a gift of nature and there is little one can do to change this, although people have inevitably tried. One old lady described how her grandmother had followed a very complicated procedure in order to do just that. She took two pieces of cotton, twice as broad as her calf, and sewed them into two bags. Sheepswool was then packed hard into the bags until they felt as solid as possible. The bags were then tied firmly around her calves before she went to bed. She had trained herself to sleep on her back to get the maximum effect from this extraordinary process and she repeated it every night. Unfortunately her grand-daughter couldn't remember if it had had any effect or not.

When Cyd Charisse was asked to what she attributed her beautiful legs she said that she alternately wore very high heels and flat shoes. This strengthened her leg muscles and improved the shape of her legs. Whether this is successful or not, it is at least simpler than the preceding method.

If you can't improve the shape of your legs you can at least improve their appearance. Hairy legs are not generally considered attractive but if the hairs are bleached they are a lot less noticeable. Shaving is the easiest method to remove unwanted hair but if not done very regularly stubbly prickly legs are the result. This is less noticeable if you remove the hair in the bath using a soapy pumice stone rubbed spirally up and down the legs, or with a piece of ultra-fine sandpaper. Both these methods can easily damage the skin and it is advisable to rub in a little almond oil after the treatment.

Obviously body packs and baths which condition the skin will also help the appearance of the legs. Goose pimples and rough skin can be removed by regular and careful use of a pumice stone or vigorous application of a loofah or sisal glove to stimulate the circulation. These gloves are often expensive to buy ready made but are very easy to make yourself. Knit or crochet a sisal rectangle twice as long and 1½ times as wide as your hand. Fold this over and sew into a bag which you can use as a bath mitt.

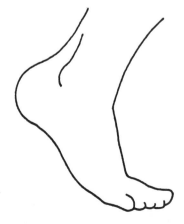

The old saying 'A woman (or a man for that matter) feels as old as her feet' is a cliche not without truth. The usual advice is of course to wear 'sensible' shoes. But if shoes are of a natural material which lets your feet breathe, and if they fit well you should get along alright. The same goes for socks, stockings and tights. Woollen or cotton socks can easily be found but who can afford pure silk tights?

The synthetic materials used in footwear increase the problem of smelly swollen feet. There are herbal footbaths which will help to regulate foot perspiration and clear the clogged pores. Steep your feet twice weekly (or more if your feet get very sweaty) in ROSEMARY infusion, decoction of OAK LEAVES or WHITE WATER LILY infusion. This last is a very effective deodorant, but for most people not readily available. BRAMBLE LEAVES (blackberry) can be found along every country lane and make a very good deodorant footbath. Boil a handful of bramble leaves for 10 minutes in 2 litres of water. Cool and bathe your feet in the warm decoction.

Tired swollen feet will benefit from a footbath in LADY'S BEDSTRAW infusion which will soothe and refresh the feet (more complicated formulae are given at the end of the chapter).

Corns, often the result of badly fitting shoes, can be treated in various ways, but ONIONS are the most frequently used remedy. Just stick a slice of raw onion over the corn with a piece of sticking plaster before going to bed. Do this every night until the corn has disappeared.

The GREATER CELANDINE is also sometimes used as a corn cure. First wash the feet in hot salt water. Then drop a little of the fresh juice or herbal tincture onto the corn and let it dry. Do this twice weekly.

Chilblains, which are caused by bad circulation, can be cured by baths in HORSE CHESTNUT decoction, prepared from the dried outer covering of the nuts and the 'conkers'. Halve the horse chestnuts and use 1 cup of conkers and outer covering to 1 litre water. It is also possible to take

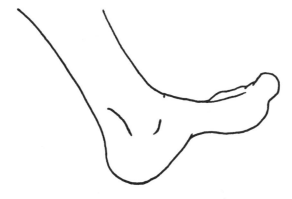

the outer covering internally to improve the circulation. Simmer 2 dessertspoonfuls dried outer covering in 1 litre water for 10 minutes. Sieve and drink 2 cups of this liquid per day. DAISY leaves are also a remedy for chilblains. Take 2 teaspoons dried daisy leaves to ½ litre water. Drink 2 dessertspoons of this infusion every day during the winter.

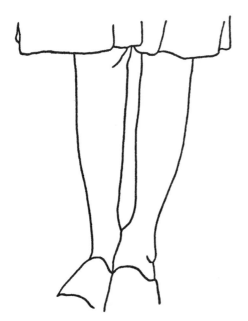

FOR TIRED FEET

10g.	Thyme
15g.	Rosemary
25g.	Peppermint
20g.	Camomile
20g.	Marjoram

Mix these herbs together. Prepare a decoction with 2 dessertspoons herbal mixture to 1 litre water. Boil for 5 minutes. Pour this into a footbath and, when it has cooled sufficiently, bathe your feet in it.

ONION CORN CURE: (a)

1 Baked onion
An equal amount of soft soap

Pulp the onion and soap together. Spread this mixture onto a piece of linen and apply it to the corn. Versions of this corn cure are to be found in many old household manuals.

ONION CORN CURE: (b)

2 slices White bread
2 slices Onion
¼ litre Natural vinegar

Put the bread and onion in a bowl. Pour the vinegar over it and leave to stand for 24 hours. Smear the corn with the bread and place a piece of onion on top of it. Secure this with a bandage, cover with a sock and leave it on overnight. A messy but effective remedy.

CHILBLAIN SALVE: (a)

Roast 2 figs in the oven. Pulverise them and mix this powder with honey. Apply to the chilblains.

CHILBLAIN SALVE: (b)

20g.   Lard
3g.   Snowdrop bulbs

Crush the bulbs into the fat with a pestle and mortar. Apply to the chilblains.

To Make a Hairy Place Bald

Take dried cats dung. Crush and mix this with strong vinegar to a pap. Smear this on often and rub it in firmly. In a few days the hairy place will become bald.
    Simon Witgeest, 1715

In order that hair may not wax, take emmets eggs, rub them up, smudge on the place, never will any hair come up there.
    The Leech Book of Bald

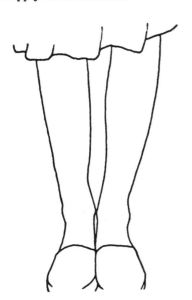

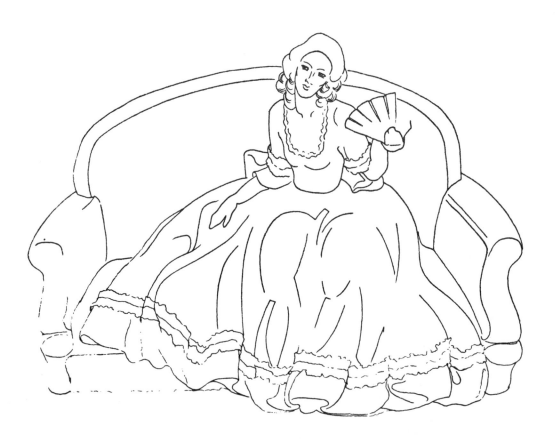

24 PERFUMES

Lavender, rose, thyme, rosemary, violets, their names make us think first of the perfumes of the flowers. The scents are pure and fine and it was often claimed by the old herbalists that the smells of flowers and herbs were remedies in themselves. Of course 'The smell of Basil is good for the heart', and 'taketh away sorrowfulness'. And who can doubt 'that the mind conceiveth a certain pleasure and recreation by smelling and handling violets' (Gerarde). In Banckes' *Herbal* we read 'Make thee a box of the wood of rosemary and smell to it and it shall preserve thy youth', a somewhat exaggerated claim, but the smell of this most loved of herbs will certainly make you feel young.

Montaigne wrote, 'Physicians might in my opinion draw more use and good from odours than they do'.

Indeed, the visitors who bring sweet-smelling flowers to a sick friend surely know better than any psychiatrist what will 'lighten the heart and cheer the mind'.

There are so many perfumes and scented products on the market that it may seem unnecessary to make your own; but it is pleasant to work with these sweet smells, and no synthetic scent can replace the freshness and clarity of natural herbs and spices.

It is, I think, as necessary to perfume your environment as your body and recipes are provided here to do both those things. Eau de Cologne and Lavender water are usually applied directly to the body but rosewater which has been used as a perfume for many centuries is perhaps best used in the bath or as a 'handwater'. For drier skins use a little essential oil of roses.

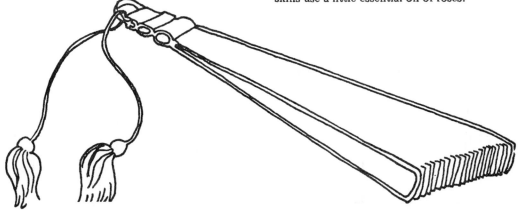

A fragrant environment can be created in many ways. Sleeping between lavender scented sheets is a delightful experience and you will carry the perfume with you all day. Just keep lavender bags in your linen drawer, the scent will penetrate sheets and pillowcases. To open a wardrobe and smell a spicy pomander is another pleasure and a bowl of pot pourri will spread a delicate fragrance through your living room. The recipes given here do not need to be followed strictly, use them as guidelines, choose your own favourite scents and mix your own 'sweet bags', pot pourris and pomanders.

The one item essential in most of these is orris powder. This is the powdered root of the iris, *Germanica, Florentina* or *Pallida* (see Herb List). These plants can be grown in this country or the powder can be obtained from chemists and herbalists.

Romantic as many of these sound they were originally developed to mask the incredibly filthy conditions in which most people lived and to ward off 'evil odours' which were thought to cause disease.

Pomanders must have been a necessity rather than a luxury in the days before refuse collection, when chamber pots were emptied from windows into the streets and washing was considered only occasionally necessary. The idea of using herbs to ward off the stench of the common folk is still found in the 'Maundy' ceremony where deserving old parishioners receive the 'Maundy money' from the hands of Her Majesty the Queen. It is a wonder that these now well-scrubbed worthies are not a little offended by the symbolism of the charming bunches of herbs held by Her Majesty and her entourage.

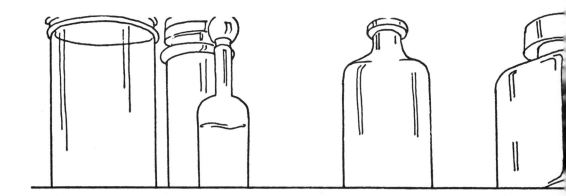

The best known way of making a pomander is to stick an orange full of cloves and then roll it in orris powder. Another sort of pomander is made with beeswax with herbs and spices kneaded into it and then rolled into balls, usually about the size of a tennis ball. These pomanders have more scope for experimentation. Use any of the herbs and spices used in the sweetbags and pot pourris.

You can also perfume your living room by throwing a few rosemary twigs on the open fire, or a handful of dried rosemary mixed with a little sugar. Those with central heating can fill the waterholder with lavender or rosemary infusion which will perfume the air as it evaporates.

POT POURRIS

Dry the flowers and herbs separately and then mix them. The powdered herbs or spices should be added last. When oils are used mix them with a little of the orris powder until they are absorbed and then add to the pot pourri. Keep the pot pourri for 1 month in a closed jar before using it.

ROSE POT POURRI

About 20	Roses
About 20	Rose geranium leaves
½ cup	Orris powder
A few drops	Rose geranium oil (quantity depends on your liking for the smell of rose geraniums)
1 flat dessertspoon	Cinnamon powder
A few pieces	Cinnamon stick
12	Cloves

Prepare as described above. From Rosemary Hemphill, *Herbs for all Seasons*.

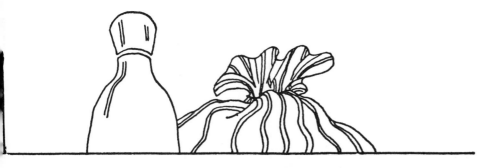

LAVENDER POT POURRI

250g. Lavender flowers (free of stalk)
20g. Dried thyme
20g. Dried mint
40g. Common salt (well dried)
10g. Ground cloves
10g. Ground caraway

Prepare as described above. From *Lotions and Potions*.

Other pot pourri herbs and flowers include pinks, orange blossom, bay leaves, mace, cedar dust, nutmeg, lemon verbena, violets, marjoram, basil, orange and lemon peel.

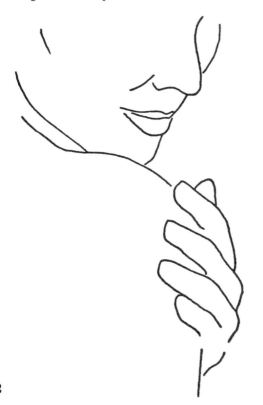

EAU DE COLOGNE: (a)

4g. Bergamot essence
4g. Citrus medica
2g. Lemon essence
2 grains Amber (Ambergris)

Put all the ingredients into a bottle and pour on them 2 litres strong spirits of wine. Keep it well corked and shake it well two or three times a day for a fortnight. Filter it through paper and put it into small bottles closely corked.

From an old recipe book, *c.* 1820. Quoted in *Lotions and Potions*.

EAU DE COLOGNE: (b)

10g. Oil of bergamot
10g. Oil of orange
10g. Oil of lemon
2g. Oil of orange blossom
2g. Oil of rosemary
1 litre Alcohol 90°

This is the formula from the French *Codex* (1437). It smells strongly of lemon but this can be softened by adding oil of roses, may, or heliotrope.

LAVENDER WATER

1 litre Spirits of wine
20g. Oil of lavender
20g. Essence of bergamot
10g. Essence of ambergris
     Musk

Combine all the ingredients. Shake the bottle well. It is better when it has been made some months.

From an old recipe book *c.* 1813. Quoted in *Lotions and Potions*.

VINAIGRE DE LAVANDE

1 litre   Lavender infusion
1/8 litre Rosewater
75g.   Vinegar

Add a little of this to your bath water for a delightful 'bouquet'.

King Edward VI's Perfume

*Take twelve spoonfuls of right red rosewater.
The weight of sexpence in fine powder of sugar
and boyle it on hot embers and coals softly, and
the house will smell as though it were full of
Roses, but you must burn the sweet Cypress wood
before, to take away the gross ayre.*
    The Queen's Closet Opened, 1655

To Make a Sweet Bag for Linnen

*Take of orris roots, sweet calamus, cypress roots,
or dried lemon peel, and dried orange peel, of each
a pound, a peck of dried roses. Make all these into
a gross powder, coriander seed four ounces, nut-
megs an ounce and a half, an ounce of cloves, ,
make all these into fine powder and mix with the
other, add musk and ambergris; then take four
large handfuls of lavender flowers dried and
rubbed; of sweet marjoram, orange leaves and
young walnut leaves, of each a handful all dried
and rubb'd: mix all together, with some bits of
cotton perfum'd with essences, and put it up into
silk bags to lay with your linnen.*
    E. Smith, *The Compleat Housewife*, 1736

All spices and herbs in different proportions can
be used to make sweet bags. Try mixed cloves,
turmeric, coriander, pine, etc.

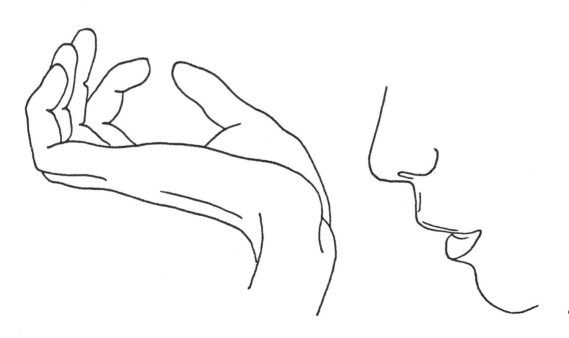

25 SLIMMING

The problem of overweight is one that concerns many men and women, both for health reasons and for the sake of their appearance. The days when voluptuous Junoesque figures and Rubens' buxom models were fashionable have passed.

An entire industry has been formed around this problem, producing slimming breads, biscuits, cakes, drinks — everything to keep or make you slim. This is, of course, nonsense. Overweight is caused by bad eating habits, or it is a serious medical problem which should be dealt with by a doctor.

Eat less, eat better, take enough exercise is the only advice anyone can give. Yet many herbalists have tried to find their own answer to weight reduction and there are various herbs which are said to be 'slimming', including CLEAVERS, FENNEL, CAMOMILE and CHICKWEED.

Culpeper mentions the use of fennel for this purpose: 'both leaves, seeds and roots thereof are used much in drink or in broth to make people more lean that are fat.'

BLADDERWRACK is also used in reducing cures, and pills made from this seaweed can be purchased in health food shops. It is said to stimulate the working of the thyroid gland and so cause the patient to lose weight.

Drinking infusions of bladderwrack has also been recommended, although it tastes revolting, and it is sometimes added to the bath water to make a 'slimming bath'. A handful of SEA SALT added to the bath water is said to have a similar, though weaker effect.

LETTUCE is also said to help to reduce weight. The theory is that lettuce takes so much energy to digest that it actually causes a loss in weight when it is eaten. However, I am afraid that only a remarkably avid lettuce eater would succeed in slimming in this way.

According to Parkinson, 'the powder of the seedes of elder first prepared in vinegar and then taken in wine halfe a dramme at a time for certaine days together is a means to abate and consume the fat flesh of a corpulent body and to keepe it lean'.

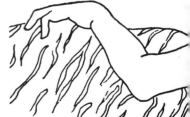

Maurice Messegue, the well-known French herbalist, sells herbal hand and foot baths, which he claims work by osmosis and will reduce weight. Most of the plants he uses have diuretic or blood purifying qualities and include ARTICHOKES, ROSEMARY, SAGE, THYME, DANDELION, BIRCH and CAMOMILE. His formula for slimming tea is given in the recipes. M. Messegue also points out that these cures are useless when the patient does not follow a balanced diet and take plenty of exercise.

The last slimming aid is SAUERKRAUT juice. A glass of this drunk before every meal will satisfy your hunger and make it easier to eat less and follow your diet. Sauerkraut juice is nourishing and blood-purifying. It can be bought ready prepared in health food shops.

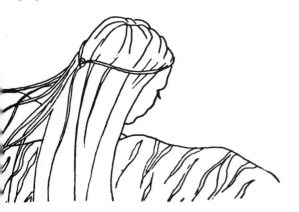

SLIMMING BATH

Bladderwrack
Dandelion
Horsetail
Camomile

Make a strong infusion, using a handful of each of these dried herbs to 2 litres water. Sieve and add the infusion to your bath. You can pinch the over-weight areas to try to reduce them.

MESSEGUE'S SLIMMING HERBAL TEA

1 handful   Cherry stalks
½ handful   Artichoke leaves
1 handful   Corn silk
1 handful   Rose petals

Infuse these herbs in 1 litre water. Drink two cups of this tea per day.

WEIGHT-REDUCING TEA

Dandelion
Fennel
Rosemary
Bladderwrack

A teaspoon of each of these herbs to ½ litre boiling water. The taste, it must be said, is most unpleasant.
From David Conway, *The Magic of Herbs.*

26 ALPHABETICAL HERB LIST

It is not the intention of this book to go into a detailed description of all the herbs and fruit mentioned. Some, such as strawberries are so well known that no description is necessary, others such as Peruvian bark and orange blossom have to be bought ready-dried from chemist, herbalist or health food shop.

The herbs listed here are all those which can be grown in Britain and the U.S.A.; read where to find them and what they look like. Most garden herbs are easy to grow and will thrive in most soils. Do not overfertilize them. A huge spreading plant will have less strength and aroma than a smaller compact one.

Most aromatic herbs like a dry sunny position. But there are plants such as lemon balm which will do well in more shady situations. Follow the instructions on your seed packet or ask the advice of your nurseryman.

Do not use chemical sprays or fertilizers on your plants, and for the very best quality herbs follow the bio-dynamic method of cultivation invented by Rudolph Steiner.

ANGELICA
(angelica officinalis)

This huge and handsome umbelliferous plant grows to a height of 4—5 feet. It grows wild in some places in the south of England but is usually cultivated in the garden. Maude Grieve in her *Modern Herbal* recommends that the fresh seed should be planted in August or September. It has been used to ward off devils and in amulets but above all in medicine as a digestive, a tonic, and as an expectorant. It is of course widely used in confectionary, its bright green candied stem being used on many cakes and sweetmeats. It is also used in the preparation of various liqueurs including Chartreuse. Here its refreshing perfume is used to sweeten the breath.

ANISE
(pimpinella anisum)

Anise is an attractive, umbelliferous annual with bright green feathery leaflets. It has white flowers and will grow to about 18 inches in height. It can be grown from seed in a sheltered, sunny position. Sew the seeds in April in a dry, light soil. They will ripen in a good summer but as this plant is a native of Egypt do not expect too much. In a wet, cold year your crop will probably fail. Anise was one of the herbs used to ward off the evil eye and it is the plant whose seeds flavour aniseed balls (and other food stuffs). We used to buy these sweets for ten a ha'penny at the corner shop. The best ones changed colour while you sucked them. Aniseed tea will ensure a good night's rest after a heavy meal. It has also been used to sweeten the breath.

BALM
(melissa officinalis)

'Balm is sovereign for the Brain, strengthening for the memory and chasing away melancoly'
   John Evelyn

Balm is a delicate attractive bushy perennial plant with soft green leaves and small pale pink flowers. It will grow to a height of about 12 inches and is an essential part of any herb garden. It will grow in any soil and thrives in half shadow. The sweet lemony fragrance of its leaves and flowers will attract bees and they are also good to use in pot pourris. According to Parkinson: *'It is a hearbe wherein bees do much delight both to have their hives rubbed therewith to keepe them together, and draw others, and for them to suck and feed upon.'*

The leaves make a delicious addition to salads and it is used in medicine for nervous conditions and fevers.

BASIL
(ocymum minimum)

This is the kitchen herb which has for centuries been grown in cottage gardens. In this country it is an annual and it can easily be grown from seed. It is best to sow the seeds in a cold frame (or in pots on the window sill) in March as it germinates slowly. It can then be planted out in May, but it can also be sown in a warm sunny spot in the garden in April. It likes a rich soil and lots of sun. Although primarily used as a pot herb, basil has been used to cure nervous disorders. Parkinson used it *'To procure a cheerfull and merry hearte'.*

BAY
(laurus nobilis)

Bay is an attractive evergreen shrub, whose aromatic leaves are widely used in the kitchen. It is the bay laurel which was used to make the wreaths of honour in ancient Greece and the Delphic priestesses chewed the leaves for their narcotic effects. In France it has been used in the treatment of rheumatism and oil of bay is used to treat sprains and bruises.

BEECH
(fagus sylvatica)

This magnificent native tree sometimes grows to 140 feet in height and 130 feet in diameter. Although its wood is not very strong and durable, it has been used for panelling and parquet flooring and other smaller articles. Beech nuts can form a valuable food for pigs and deer, but they are said to be poisonous for horses. The wood tar is used to treat bronchitis and various skin diseases.

BETONY
(betonica officinalis)

This attractive woodland plant grows to about 1 foot in height. The flowers are reddish purple and labiate, forming dense heads at the top of the stems. The leaves are sparse, oblong and grow in pairs. Betony has always been associated with magic and was considered extremely effective in driving away evil spirits. Medically, betony was used as a panacea by herbalists all over Europe but it is nowadays mainly used to treat nervous complaints and headaches.

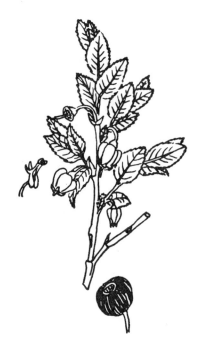

BIRCH
(betula alba)

The Silver Birch is a dainty lady,
She wears a satin gown;
  E. Nesbit

'The lady of the woods' is a beautiful and elegant tree with its silver stem and graceful branches. It is used in many skin preparations and medicinally for fevers (the inner bark). A preparation of the leaf sap is diuretic. Birch syrup is a well known tonic, said to keep you young.

BLADDERWRACK
(fucus vesiculosis)

A common sea weed. Coarse yellow or brownish green in colour. It is easily recognisable by its oval air vesicles which form the characteristic 'bladders' with which many generations of children have amused themselves on the beach, bursting them between their fingers.

Commercially bladderwrack forms an excellent potash-rich fertilizer. It was once used in the manufacture of iodine, and has been an ingredient in rheumatism cures and in oils for the treatment of sprains and bruises. Today it is best known for its weight-reducing properties.

BILBERRY
(vaccinium myrtillus)

This well known herb which grows in woods and on moorland is best known for its delicious dark blue berries used in tarts and jams. It is a low woody plant with small pointed leaves. In cosmetics it is used for its astringent proprieties. Medically it is used in the treatment of dysentery and diarrhoea, and is sometimes used to treat ulcers.

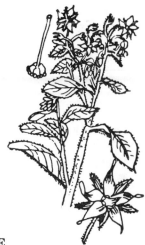

BORAGE
(borago officinalis)

I borage,
Bring alwaies courage.
    Anon.

This beautiful herb with its downy leaves and pendulous, sky blue, star-shaped flowers was used by many of the old herbalists:

'To make the mind glad'
    Gerarde

'To repress the fulginous uproar of dusky melan-cholie'
    Bacon

It is a hardy annual which will seed itself and come up year after year in the same place, if it has enough sun.

In medicine it is used to cool fevers and for its diuretic qualities. Borage also has emollient and purifying qualities which are useful in the treatment of skin complaints.

BRAMBLE
(rubus fruticosus)

Her apples were swart blackberries,
Her currants, pods o'broom;
Her wine was dew of the wild white rose,
Her book a church-yard tomb.
    John Keats, *Meg Merrilees*

The prickly bramble (or blackberry) needs no description. How familiar this plant has been through the ages is shown by the amount of extra-ordinary folk customs associated with it. Children who suffered from a hernia condition used to be passed under an arch of blackberry which was rooted at both ends. It was said to be a certain cure.

In America the bramble could forecast a good harvest:

'if the bramble bloom in June
harvest bounty follows soon'

There are several biblical references to this plant and there is a tradition that it was the burning bush which appeared to Moses.

The fruits which are rich in minerals have been used to treat anaemia. Tea made from the leaves will cure diarrhoea and make a soothing cough remedy. The leaves have deodorant qualities and were used in gynaecology.

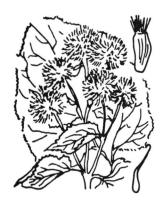

CAMOMILE
(Anthemis nobilis)

I am sorry to say that Peter was not very well during the evening. His mother put him to bed, and made some camomile tea; and she gave a dose of it to Peter!

'One tablespoonful to be taken at bed time.'
Beatrix Potter, *The Tale of Peter Rabbit.*

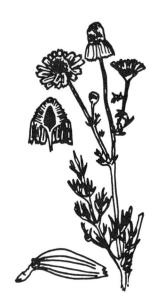

BURDOCK
(arctium lappa)

This splendid member of the thistle family grows on damp wastelands throughout England. It can reach 3 to 4 feet in height and has large, broad leaves and round purple flower heads. The prickly seedheads attach themselves to everything. Celia and Rosalind had to contend with them:

Rosalind: How full of briars is this working day world!

Celia: They are but burrs, cousin, thrown upon thee in holiday foolery. If we walk not in trodden paths our very petticoats will catch them.

The part of this plant used in medicine and cosmetics is the root, which is an excellent blood-purifier and is used to cure various skin diseases.

This little daisy-like flower has bright green feathery leaves and can grow to about 12 inches high.

It grows on wasteland, in cornfields and along the wayside. The flowers appear from July to September and are borne on a single slender stem. It prefers dry sandy ground. If this plant does not grow wild in your area, try planting it in a sunny position. The seeds can be sown in May. The double camomile in particular makes a very attractive garden flower.

It is its scent which makes this plant so easily recognisable. It is strongly aromatic and releases its perfume when crushed or walked over. Camomile lawns are coming back into fashion and camomile seats, a common feature of old herb gardens, may also regain their popularity. It was considered very beneficial to health and spirit to sit on these fragrant seats and inhale the perfume.

All the old herbalists give long lists of the uses of camomile. Parkinson says:

Camomile is put to divers and sundry uses, both for pleasure and profit, both for sick and sound, in bathing to comfort and strengthen the sound and to ease pains in the diseased'.

Camomile tea, although unpleasant to taste, will soothe stomach cramps (like Peter Rabbit's) and is an effective sedative. It is one of the most useful cosmetic herbs and is used for various purposes throughout this book.

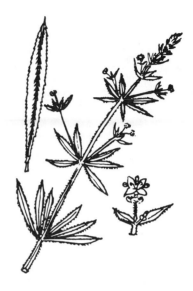

CHICKWEED
(stellaria media)

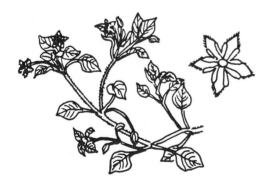

A small but persistent weed, chickweed trails along the ground. It has small, light green, egg-shaped leaves and delicate star-like flowers. Birds love it and it is an excellent tonic for them. Herbalists use it in ointments to soothe inflammations and ulcers. In this book it is used in a face lotion.

CLEAVERS
(galium aparine)

This is an easily recognisable hedgerow plant and is also known as goose-grass. It climbs up through the hedgerows in dense masses, clinging to everything it touches including our clothes, which makes it a favourite with children. The leaves are long and pointed, growing round the stem in whorls. The greenish-white star-shaped flowers are rather insignificant and are not as well known as the clinging, globular seed vessels. The roots have been used to make a red dye and it is even said that birds which eat the plant get red bones. Parkinson also says that country folk used cleavers as a strainer *'to clear their milke from straws, haires and any other thing that falleth into it'.*

Cleavers are used for many different medical purposes, most commonly for skin diseases, scurvy and urinary problems. It makes an excellent hair rinse, due to its effect on the scalp. **81**

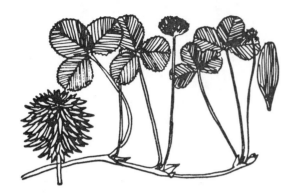

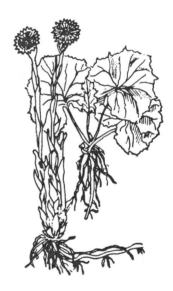

CLOVER

*Why and whither and how? for barley and rye
are not clover:
Neither are straight lines curves: yet over is under
and over.*
    Algernon Charles Swinburne, *The Higher
    Pantheism in a Nutshell*

WHITE CLOVER
(trifolium repens)

This well known wayside and meadow flower is
too well known to need any description. The
flowers are used to purify the blood.

RED CLOVER
(trifolium pratense)

This used to be widely used as a fodder crop but
will not grow on land fertilized with nitrates and
is now seldom grown. The bees prefer the white
variety.

Our forefathers used red clover to treat bronchitis
and whooping cough, and to make into the red
clover lip & wound salve.

82

COLTSFOOT
(tussilago farfara)

This cheerful yellow flower which covers waste
land in early February and heralds the coming of
Spring, is in fact a very useful herb and in France
was used as the sign to indicate the apothecaries'
shops. It owes its name to its large 'hoof' shaped
leaves which appear after the flowers have died
away. An excellent cough medicine can be
prepared from the fresh leaves and juice and the
dried leaves are used in herbal tobacco to relieve
asthma. The plant is emollient and is used in face
creams and hair lotions.

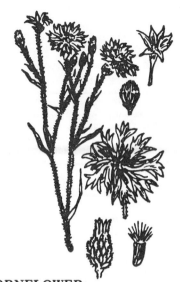

CORNFLOWER
(centaurea cyanus)

How appropriate it is that this intensely blue flower should symbolise clarity. Before chemical sprays were so widely used it did indeed bloom in and along cornfields, together with the scarlet poppy, but that beautiful sight has now become rare although the cornflower can still be found on commons and waysides. It is an easy plant to grow in the garden. Plant the seeds in the spring in a sunny border and the flowers will be ready to harvest in August. The flower is used in eyewaters and to give colour to pot pourris. It is popular in cosmetics for its softening qualities.

COWSLIP
(primula veris)

The cowslip is one of our most attractive spring flowers. The wrinkled oval leaves form a rosette on the ground from which rises a single stalk which carries the flower head. The clear yellow flowers are bell shaped and form an umbel at the top of the stalk. This plant grows in damp meadows. The cowslip flowers are lightly narcotic and have been widely used in country remedies to strengthen the nerves, relieve headaches and combat sleeplessness. It is a cosmetic herb which has been used since early times in creams and lotions to prevent wrinkles. Primroses are used in the same way but their active ingredients are much weaker.

DAISY
(bella perennis)
'The Day's Eye' [old English name]

This very common but attractive little flower had a wide reputation as a wound herb. It is even said that chewing the leaves will cure an ulcerated mouth. Gerarde called it 'bruisewort' and recommended it 'For all kinds of aches and pains'. Daisy water is a very old beauty lotion mentioned in many herbals and manuals.

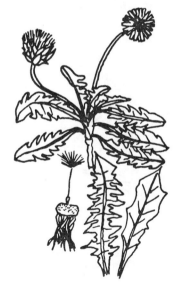

DANDELION
(taraxacum officinale)

This 'gardener's curse and children's 'clock' is considered a table delicacy in France and Italy where the bleached leaves are eaten in salads.

It is a very handsome plant with its 'yellow head which beams like the sun itself' (Melly Uyldert) and its jagged leaves like the 'dents de lion' which gives it its name.

The dandelion makes a tonic recommended by all herbalists to stimulate the entire organism. It is diuretic and called 'pis en lit' (wet the bed) in France. This plant is part of the Spring cure which will in itself help to clear the skin, and it is used externally to treat spots and pimples.

the deep shiny black berries. The young stems are hollow and have often been used to make musical pipes or pop guns for small boys.

The legends I have quoted about the elder tree are but a few of the hundreds of tales of its magical powers, but its practical uses are also innumerable. The leaves are said to keep away insects. The wood is used for making small and fine objects; the flowers for face lotions, vinegar, wine and fritters; elderberries for wine, to colour inferior wine (afterwards to be sold at a higher price), for jams and to make elderberry rob, a syrup which makes a most effective cold remedy.

The bark is used in emollient ointments and homeopathic asthma cures. The root was, in ancient times, used as a purgative.

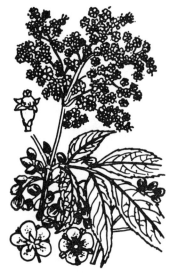

ELDER
(sambucus nigra)

The elder, so the old stories say, was the tree used for the cross of Calvary. Judas is said to have hung himself from one of its branches. And long before the birth of Christ it was planted near human habitation to keep the inhabitants safe from evil spirits.

The tree is best known for its fragrant, flat-topped bunches of white flowers which are followed by

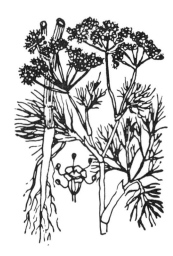

FENNEL
(foeniculum vulgare)

Above the lowly plants in towers,
The fennel, with its yellow flowers,
And in an earlier age than ours
Was gifted with the wondrous power
Lost vision to restore.
        H. W. Longfellow

What a beautiful and graceful plant fennel is. It can grow four to five feet in height and has the most delicate bright green feathery foliage in the garden. The flat umbels of yellow flowers attract innumerable bees and nectar loving insects. It is a joy to watch the ceaseless activity around this fragrant plant on a warm day in July or August. Fennel is a perennial and will grow easily from seed in a sunny position. It has been used to keep away both devils and fleas:

Plant fennel
Near a kennel.

says an old rhyme. It is good advice. As Longfellow pointed out, fennel seed tea was used by the Red Indians to restore their sight. It was an ingredient of 'gripe water' and was used to make a cough syrup. In the kitchen it is mainly used with fish and in the south of France fennel is displayed on every market fish stall to keep the fish 'fresh' — although it in fact just disguises the smell by masking it with its own sweet aromatic perfume.

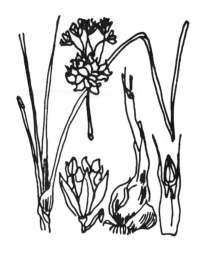

FUMITORY
(fumaria officinalis)
'Smoke of the Earth'

This is a small grey-green plant with angular branching stems and fine, much divided leaves. It flowers in midsummer and its very pale pink flowers growing as a terminal spike, also add to its 'smokey' appearance. There is a legend which says that this herb was born from vapours rising out of the earth. It has in ancient times been burned so that its smoke would drive away evil spirits. Fumitory is used to treat liver disorders, in skin tonics and as a skin bleaching agent. The flowers can be made into a yellow dye for wool.

GARLIC
(allium sativum)

This remarkable, pungent plant is usually bought at the greengrocer to flavour food, but it can be grown quite easily and successfully by any gardener. Separate a bulb of garlic into cloves and plant these early in the Spring in a moist, well fertilised flower bed. They should be ready to harvest in August. It is good to plant garlic between rose trees as it will help to keep the roses free from disease and the two plants have a good influence upon each other. Some even say that the garlic makes the roses smell sweeter!

Many legends and miracle cures have been attributed to this plant. Dracula fans will be aware of its anti-vampire qualities, but may not have heard this old Muslim legend: when Satan left the garden of Eden after his successful temptation of Eve, garlic sprang from his left footprint and onion from his right one. It is nice to know we have something to thank Satan for.

Garlic is nature's antibiotic. Its very strong antiseptic constituents have worked many cures. It will help to prevent colds and even hardening of the arteries. It can be worked into ointments to relieve asthma and tightness of the chest and will purify the blood. Caucasian peasants have attributed their longevity to a diet containing considerable quantities of yoghurt and garlic. As if all this was not enough, garlic is also said to stimulate hair growth and is used in hair lotions.

GREATER CELANDINE
(chelidonium majus)

This is the true celandine, a herbacious perennial which grows from 1½ to 3 feet in height. It has leaves resembling those of the buttercup in shape but paler in colour. The flowers are bright yellow and four-petalled. The whole plant has a strong, unpleasant smell emitting from the bright orange sap in which it abounds. The old name for this plant is swallow wort. Parkinson quotes Pliny saying 'it tooke that name from the swallowes that cured their young ones eyes that were hurt, with bringing this herb, and putting it to them'. A most extraordinary tale.

Under the doctrine of signatures the greater celandine was used to cure jaundice and in this case there is some evidence to support the claim. It is also used to cure scrofulous diseases. The plant contains poisonous substances and it is not advisable to experiment with it. The juice is a powerful irritant and is used to remove corns.

GROUNDSEL
(senecio vulgaris)

This ragged inconspicuous little weed, with its small yellow flowers makes an excellent tonic for cage birds. It has been widely used as a mild purgative and is said to ease menstrual pains Groundsel is also an old folk remedy for chapped hands.

HAWTHORN
(crataegus oxyacantha)

The hawthorn or May is a common hedgerow tree with its white blossoms and bright red berries in the autumn. The children's saying that if you pick the May blossoms you will wet the bed is not without foundation as the hawthorn is a diuretic. It is used as a cardiac tonic and as an astringent.

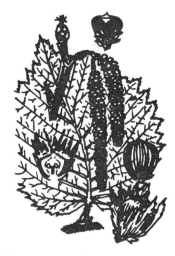

HAZEL
(corylus avellana)

A magic tree, planted around Red Riding Hood's grandmother's house and Cinderella's mother's grave. There are so many legends about this small graceful tree with its yellow catkins in spring and its delicious nuts in the autumn that it is impossible to quote them all in this book. The nuts are said to be good for heart patients and for anaemia. The leaves are astringent and are used in face lotions.

HONEYSUCKLE
(lonicera periclymenum)

This fragrant climbing plant can be found in
gardens, woods and hedgerows all over the
country. It climbs to 30 feet in height and
produces delicate trumpet-shaped pinkish yellow
flowers with a delicious perfume. The syrup made
from honeysuckle flowers is used to treat asthma,
bronchitis and other diseases of the respiratory
organs.

HORSERADISH
(amoracia rusticana)

Anyone who enjoys eating horseradish sauce
should obtain a root to plant in the garden. Put
the root at least a foot deep in rich, well fertilised
ground. The plant will grow three to four feet in
height and has very attractive feathery leaves and
white flowers with a pleasant, peppery smell. It is
possible to dig out part of the root for use without
damaging the plant as a whole. Horseradish is
strongly diuretic and antiseptic. It was used as a
remedy for worms and is still frequently applied
on a poultice to ease congestion of the chest and
lungs. Cosmetically it is used as a bleaching agent.

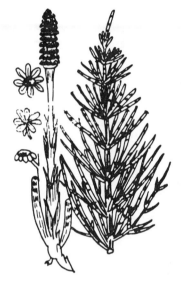

HORSETAIL
(equisetum arvense)

This fascinating plant group, the *equisetacea*, is a
left over from the carboniferous period when
plants of this family dominated the vegetation.
They are now microscopic representations of what
they once were. Their stems are erect, jointed and
brittle. The fertile stems are unbranched and bear
a cone-like catkin on top. But it is the infertile
ones which give the plant its name, with their
whorls of stiff 'bristles' which become smaller
towards the top giving the plant its characteristic
'horsetail shape'. In medicine it is used for its
diuretic and astringent qualities. It is used as an
astringent in various lotions and for fingernails. 87

IRIS
(iris florentina, iris germanica, iris pallida)

These three irises are those used to make the violet scented 'orris powder' so frequently used in sweet bags and pot pourris. The powder is made from the dried rhizome of the plant which takes 2—3 years to mature. These iris make very attractive garden flowers. The *iris pallida* has pale blue flowers, the *germanica* a deeper blue flower and the *florentina* large white ones. They will flourish in a normal well fertilised border and do not require excessive moisture. In Italy these iris are grown commercially and orris powder can be obtained from chemists and herbalists.

JASMINE
(jasminium grandiflora)

This is the jasmine cultivated for its perfume in the region of Cannes and Grasse. It is grown as an erect bush and has a delicious perfume. The dried flowers can be bought at some herbalists.

(jasminium officinale)

This is a hardy climber with white flowers which bloom throughout the summer. It is a common garden plant and will grow well on a sunny, south-facing wall. The flowers are suitable to use in pot pourris and sweet bags, although their fragrance is fainter than that of *grandiflora*. Jasmine symbolises love and has frequently been used in 'love potions'.

JUNIPER
(juniperus communis)

The juniper is a small coniferous shrub 4—6 feet high. It is best known for its fragrant black berries used to flavour gin. Oil of juniper is said to be a cure for indigestion, and is strongly diuretic. Sheep who eat the berries of this shrub apparently cure themselves of dropsy!

88

LADY'S BEDSTRAW
(galium verum)

Lady's bedstraw has clusters of bright yellow flowers growing towards the top of very upright stems. The leaves are very fine and narrow growing in whorls of 6—8. It grows to about 2 feet high and prefers dry positions near the sea. It flowers in late summer. It has been frequently used as both a red and yellow dye, the roots producing the red colour and the stem and leaves the yellow. This herb also has the name 'cheese rennet' because of its use in cheese making. The plant is not so widely used in medicine as it used to be although it is still considered a cure for some diseases of the bladder. In this book it is used in a foot bath. Gerarde preferred to use it in an ointment 'for anointing the weary traveller'.

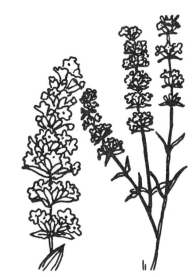

LAVENDER
(lavendula)

Lavender's blue dilly dilly
Lavender's green
When you are king dilly dilly,
I will be queen.

English lavender *(lavendula vera)* is the most fragrant of the lavenders. It is obviously an essential part of any herb garden. It can be grown from seed but this perennial plant is more often propagated by cuttings and layering. Plants are easy to obtain from any nursery. Lavender likes a sunny position and a light soil. For a garden curiosity, try to find a plant of the rare white variety. It is less hardy but has a very delicate perfume. All lavenders are usually grown for their perfume, or as Parkinson puts it,

'Lavender, is almost wholly spent with us, for to perfume linnen apparell, gloves and leather and the dryed flowers to comfort and dry up the moisture of a cold braine'.

But oil of lavender is a stimulant and restorative. It will relieve headaches caused by fatigue and is lightly antiseptic.

LEMON VERBENA
(lippia citridora)

This shrub originates from Chile and Peru but is often found in this country, planted in sheltered gardens. It is deciduous and grows to about twelve feet in height. The mauve flowers appear in August but it is the long pointed leaves which retain the sweet, characteristic perfume, so invaluable in sweet bags and pot pourris. Medically it is used to calm a dyspeptic stomach.

LILY
(lilium)

A lily of a day
Is fairer far in May
Although it fall and die that night
It was the plant and flower of light.
    (from an ode by Ben Johnson)

It is said that in this time of sexual freedom and obsession with bodily pleasures, the lily has become unpopular, since it has always symbolised purity and virginity. It is a spiritual plant, far removed from present day materialism. This theory may be rather far-fetched, but it is true that these beautiful flowers are no longer the pride of our gardens, as they were in the seventeenth and eighteenth centuries. For most people today a lily is the rather stiff white arum lily, seen at funerals and in church at Easter. Many other attractive members of this family with their Chinese lantern shapes and various colours will grow well in most well fertilized gardens, if they are planted deep enough to protect them from severe frosts. Lilies are said to purify the blood and have for centuries been used to treat gynaecological complaints. The oil is used to cure ear ache and heal skin diseases

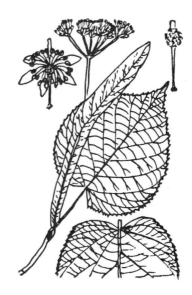

LIME TREE
(tilia europaea)

One of our most beautiful and fragrant trees. The lime will grow to 140 feet in height. With its clear green heart-shaped leaves, well proportioned branches and refreshing perfume it will 'rejoice the   **89** heart to look upon it' (Melly Uyldert). The wood of this tree has been widely used for carving, but in this book we are concerned with the small white or yellowish flowers which are so widely used to make tea. In France no household would be without 'tilleul' which is drunk as soon as someone feels slightly off-colour for its refreshing and soothing effect. It will lubricate a dry throat and calm a nervous stomach. As a lotion it will refresh the skin and condition your hair.

LOVAGE
(levesticum officinale)

'The whole plant and every part of it smelleth strongly and aromatically and of a hot, sharpe, biting taste'
    Parkinson

This old English herb with its attractive name has a hollow stalk and rough dark green leaves, rather like an unbleached celery. As Parkinson says it is very aromatic, with a more intense, more spicy scent than celery. It was previously widely used as a pot herb. It can be easily grown from seed in a sunny place. Lovage is used as a tonic, to drink, bathe in or apply externally. It has also had aphrodisiac properties attributed to it.

LUPIN
(lupinus perenis)

A familiar garden flower with tall spikes of blue, pink and white flowers. It was, surprisingly in view of its looks, a plant associated with witches who used the seeds for worming cattle. Its uses were wide and at a famous dinner party in Hamburg lupin enthusiast Dr. Thomas fed his guests entirely with dishes containing lupin flowers, seeds, oils and extracts, served on a lupin fibre tablecloth. There were lupin paper place cards and in the cloakrooms lupin soap was provided for the guests to wash their hands. Parkinson mentions the use of ground lupin seeds to make a complexion cream 'mingled with the gall of a goate and some juyce of limons'.

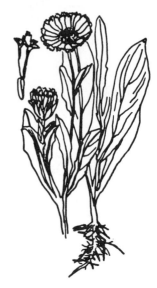

MARIGOLD
(calendula officinalis)

'The Marigold that goes to bed wi'th' sun. And with him rises weeping'
    A Winter's Tale

This attractive abundant garden flower is often today considered too unsophisticated for those immaculate gardens filled with dahlias, chrysanthemums and hybrid roses. But it was loved by the old herbalists and considered an excellent 'pot herb'. Gerarde thought 'no broths are well made without dried Marigold'. Calendula salve is widely used on the continent to heal small wounds, and stings. In cosmetics it is used for its astringent and disinfectant qualities.

MARJORAM
(origanum majorana)

This excellent pot herb is one of the few herbs whose fragrance increases when dried. It is therefore a very useful herb to grow in the garden in some quantity. It will grow well in a light soil in a sunny position. Sow the seeds in March—April. It will grow into a busy plant about 8 inches high with little white labiate flowers. Marjoram is a perennial plant, but after 3 years the flavour decreases so it is wise to have new plants ready. Medically marjoram is antiseptic and good for the stomach and has also been used to treat bronchial disorders and coughs. It also played a role in treating the vapours, used in the same way as smelling salts.

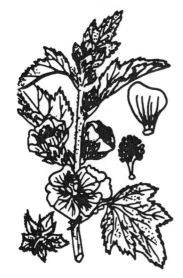

MARSH-MALLOW
(althaea officinalis)

This tall plant (3—4ft high) grows in salt marshes, in damp meadows and ditches. It is found locally in England. The leaves are 3—4 inches long with five lobes and serrated edges. The flowers are pale pink with five petals resembling those of the hollyhock, which is a member of the same family. These are paler than those of the common mallow, and the stems of the marsh-mallow are hairy. It is possible to use the common mallow in place of the marsh-mallow although its active qualities are not so strong. It can be raised from

seed in a damp corner of the garden. The root is used in cosmetics for its emollient qualities. It is used in medicine to soothe alimentary inflammations and to treat coughs, colds and bronchitis.

MEADOWSWEET
(spiraea ulmaria)

'Queen Elizabeth of famous memorie did more desire meadowsweet than any other sweete herbe to strewe her chambers withall.'
   Parkinson

A beautiful flower which grows in damp meadows and along the banks of quiet streams. Its sweet scent perfumes the summer air and its bunches of creamy white flowers are a delight to see. It has feathery white foliage and tall dark stems 2—4 feet high. The herb has often been used in beer making and health giving drinks for invalids. It is also a cure for diarrhoea. Meadowsweet was one of the sacred plants of the Druids. It is here included in a depurative drink to clear the skin.

MINT
(mentha)

There are so many members of the mint family, both wild and cultivated, that it is impossible to go into a detailed description of them here.

Peppermint *(mentha piperita)* is perhaps the best known as this is the mint sort so widely used in the kitchen and to flavour sweets. Dried peppermint also makes a pleasant cooling tea which is very good for dyspepsia and flatulence.

In this book however we are mainly concerned with the refreshing stimulating aromas of these plants and it is a matter of individual preference which members of the mint family you personally find most pleasing.

91

MISTLETOE
(viscum album)

This parasitic and sacred plant of the Druids, under which we kiss at Christmas, has also medical and cosmetic uses. In 1720 Sir John Colbatch published a pamphlet on the 'Treatment of Epilepsy by mistletoe' and it was long used for this purpose. Anthroposophic doctors still hold this herb in high esteem. In this book it is used, much more prosaically, to treat pimples.

MUGWORT
(artemisia vulgaris)

'The mother of the herbs'

This large aromatic plant grows up to 3—4 ft in height. The stem is woody, reddish and grooved. The leaves are jagged, dark green on the upper surface and white and downy on the lower surface. The small flowers vary from yellow to red in colour and appear during the summer months.

This herb has been used in folk medicine and magic for generations. It is sometimes known as St. John's Plant and on St. John's Day in Limburg a cross was made from the roots and thrown into the fire to ward off evil. It has been used to drive away devils since Anglo-Saxon times and was often worn as an amulet. On the continent people going on a long journey would put a piece of mugwort in each shoe to ease their steps and hasten their return. Medically it is used as a mild stimulant and is good for women during the menopause. It is also a purifying herb and is therefore used in drinks to clear the skin.

OAK
(quercus robur)

The English Oak is a sturdy fellow
He gets his green coat late.
  E. Nesbit, Our Trees in Spring

The oak is perhaps the most valuable of all our trees. The strength, durability and beauty of its wood are well known. It is perhaps its remarkable longevity which has fascinated people and given rise to the innumerable superstitions and stories told of it. The Druids held their religious ceremonies in oak groves and King Arthur's round table was a slice of an enormous oak trunk. Acorns were used for feeding swine and there were special laws relating to this which persisted throughout the medieval period. It will be remembered that Pooh's friend Piglet existed on a diet of 'haycorns'. The oak was used medically for its astringent properties and the leaves are said to be an effective deodorant.

PARSLEY
(apium petroselinum)

This common kitchen herb must surely be grown in every herb garden. It is notoriously slow to germinate as according to an old French story it must go seven times to find the devil and return to its place before starting to grow and then it will only do so if the gardener is an honest man (or woman). It is therefore wise to plant the first crop of seeds in February. They should then return from their wanderings in time to sprout by Easter. Parsley is very rich in minerals and trace elements and should be eaten as much as possible. A curative oil known as apiol is extracted from the seeds. The whole plant makes an excellent tonic and the root is diuretic.

PENNYROYAL
(mentha pulegium)

The smallest member of the mint family, penny-royal creeps along the ground and has small, grey-green, round-oval leaves. The red-purple-blue flowers occur at the axil of the leaves and flower from July until August. Pennyroyal is perhaps the most pungent of the mint family. It was considered conducive to good health to have it hanging in the bedroom and it is used as a blood-purifier.

Our garden mints, peppermint *(mentha piperata)* and spearmint *(mentha viridis)*, have a finer fragrance and are on the whole more suited to use in pot pourri and sweet bags than pennyroyal.

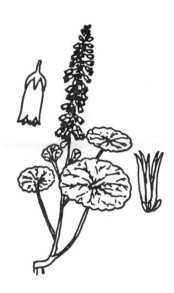

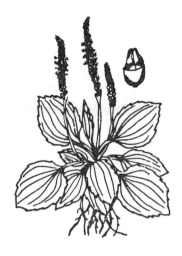

PENNYWORT
(cotyledon umbilicus)
(umbilicus rupestris)

This is an easily recognisable but not so well known plant. It can be found in sheltered places along walls and hedges. The leaves are thick and round. They are light green and the upper side is slightly hollowed. The edges of the leaves are serrated. The flowers are bell shaped and whitish green in colour and grow round the long stem which grows to a length of about 9 inches. The plant is used as an antiseptic, and in mixtures to cure spots and pimples.

PLANTAIN
(plantago major)

A familiar weed which grows along every wayside. It has broad round leaves and long stems ending in the flower head which later bears the well known brown seeds. Plantain is an ancient plant and we find it included in this Anglo-Saxon recipe for 'Flying Venom':

'Take a handful of hammer wort and a handful of maythe and a handful of waybroad [plantain] and roots of water dock, seek those which will float, and one eggshell full of clean honey, then take clean butter, let him who will help to work up the salve melt it thrice, let one sing a mass over the warts, before they are put together and the salve is wrought up'

Nowadays plantain leaves are used to cool fevers, as a wound herb and in making an effective cough medicine.

PRIMROSE
(primula vulgaris)

This well known spring flower with its five pale
yellow petals and wrinkled leaves, is closely
related to the cowslip and has similar medical
properties, although the cowslip is considered to
be more powerful, and has been more widely used
by herbalists. Pliny, however thought highly of this
flower and used it to treat muscular complaints.

QUINCE
(cydonia vulgaris)

This ancient tree is no longer as popular as it once
was. Its history goes back into the mists of time.
What is certain is that the Greeks, and later the
Romans, thought highly of this fruit and it
features in many wall paintings. Recipes for quince
jellies and marmalades can be found in mediaeval
recipe books. It is a small, many-branched tree
which takes on fantastic twisted forms as it
becomes older. Quince syrup is prepared to treat
diarrhoea and the quince pip slime is used in
throat diseases, to treat diarrhoea and dysentery
and in soothing creams and lotions.

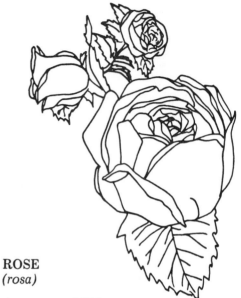

ROSE
(rosa)

Are you cross? Pick a rose
Put it on your hat
You'll soon feel glad.

It is quite unnecessary to go into descriptions of
this most sung and written about flower. But rosewater is such a common ingredient in cosmetics it
is necessary to describe exactly what this is.
'The British Pharmacopoeia directs that it shall be
prepared by mixing distilled rosewater of
commerce obtained mostly from *Rosa damascena*
but also from *Rosa centifolia* and other species,
with twice its volume of distilled water
immediately before use'. (Maude Grieve, *A
Modern Herbal*). However for our homemade
creams it is possible to use a herbal infusion of
fresh damask roses.

True oil or attar of roses is produced by distilling
roses and collecting the small amount of oil
released during this process. Bulgarian attar of
roses is considered the best as they distill the rose
water several times, collecting the oil after each
distillation. 4000 kilos of roses distilled in this way
give 1 kilo of attar of roses.

In France 10,000 kilos of roses are needed to produce 1 kilo of oil but the distilled water is sold separately as rosewater and has only one distillation. It will be clear from this that attar of roses is very expensive and although it is an ingredient of true cold creams (even 2 drops will make a difference to its quality), there will be few people who will feel inclined to use such a costly item.

For pot pourris Maude Grieve suggests *Rosa gallica* and *Rosa dentifolia*. There are many hybrids from these varieties and it should not be difficult to select some suitable for your garden.

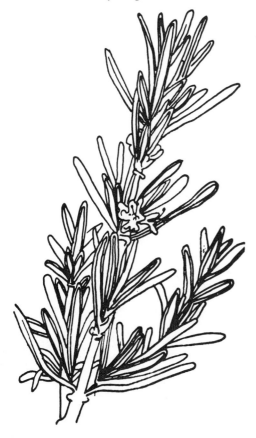

ROSEMARY
(rosmarinus officinalis)

Rosemary Rosemary
Is your name
Dew of the sea
Is in Latin, the same.
    Anon.

Rosemary must be the most loved of all the true herbs. The old herbalists sang its praises and wrote long descriptions of its good qualities. It is a beautiful plant. A shrubby herb which will grow 2—3 feet high in this country. The leaves are hard linear and very dark green. The small flowers are a very beautiful shade of soft blue. The aromatic perfume is rich and spicy.

It will grow in a warm light soil and likes a very sheltered sunny position. There is a manuscript in the British Museum sent by the Countess of Hainault to her daughter Queen Philippa in which she describes all the virtues of this plant and tells the old story that rosemary will never exceed the height of man while he is on earth. Another legend attributes the blue colour of flowers to the time the Virgin Mary hung her robe on a rosemary bush. The white flowers have from that day taken the colour of Mary's cloth.

The uses to which rosemary was put are too many to quote here but in the Grete Herbal we read:

'For weyknesse of ye brayne. Against weyknesse of the brayne and coldnesse thereof, sethe rosemaria in wyne and lete the pacyent receye the smoke at his nose and keep his heed warme.'

Rosemary has often been said to 'strengthen the memory' and has been used to symbolise remembrance in love and in death. It is used to cure headaches but is nowadays principally used in hair lotions and shampoos.

95

SAGE
(salvia officinalis)

He that would live for aye
Must eat sage in May.

Sage is a common kitchen herb with a rich,
pungent, spicy scent. It is a shrubby plant with
grey-green leaves and blue-purple labiate flowers.
It is usually bought as a small plant from a nursery,
but this perennial can be grown from seed in
sheltered positions. Sage likes a warm, dry bed and
will repay careful treatment by the delightful
perfume that wafts through the garden every time
the sun shines on it. It is advisable to replant with
new sage plants every three to four years.

Sage tea makes an excellent gargle for a sore throat
and for weak gums. It is a cooling drink during
fevers and has purifying qualities. The red variety,
with its red coloured leaves, is a most effective hair
dye, but the ordinary grey-green leaves will also
darken the hair.

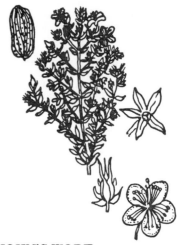

ST JOHN'S WORT
(hypericum perforatum)

This magic herb used to be called 'Faga
Daemonum', as it was believed that one smell of
its pungent scent would send demons back to hell.
It is a perennial with erect stems which branch
towards the top; the bright yellow flowers appear
at the top of these stems. The leaves are pale green
and oblong, with small spots which can be seen when
the plant is held up to the light. These are the oil
glands. St. John's wort is used medically for
pulmonary complaints.

SAVORY
(satureia hortensis)

Summer savory is the herb which is used in this
book. It is a common garden herb which will grow
from seed in sunny positions. Sow the seeds in
April. They will need thinning out later in the
Spring. Savory is a hardy annual which grows to a
foot high. The mauve labiate flowers appear in
July. The leaves are small and linear, the stems
hairy. Savory is an old pot herb and has calming
and warming virtues. It will soothe insect stings
and skin irritations.

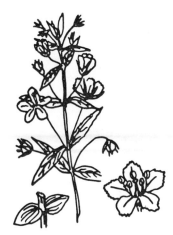

SCARLET PIMPERNEL
(anagallis arvensis)

No heart can think, no tongue can tell
The virtues of the pimpernell
    Anon.

This attractive little plant has square stems and small smooth leaves arranged in pairs. The small five petalled scarlet flower is only visible in bright weather and as soon as the day clouds over it shuts tightly, forecasting rain. The pimpernel was at one time considered a universal panacea and is still used to treat some brain diseases. It has for centuries been used as a cosmetic to clear the skin.

SELF-HEAL
(prunella vulgaris)

When little elves have cut themselves
Or mouse has hurt her tail,
Or froggie's arm has come to harm
This herb will never fail.
    Cicely M. Barker, *Flower fairies of the*
    wayside.

This small but valued herb is recognisable by its 'ear' of purple labiate flowers crowded together at the top of the stem. The rather hairy oval leaves grow off the short stems lower down the square central stem. The plant can be found on waste ground all over the British Isles. The name tells of its uses, in both ancient and modern times it has been used as a wound herb. Its astringent action is equally effective internally and externally.

SHEPHERD'S PURSE
(capsella bursa-pastoris)

This innocuous little weed with its jagged leaves and small whitish flowers is usually identified by its triangular seed pods, the 'shepherd's purses' which give it its name. An unimportant plant to look at but one of the most potent herbs to stop haemorrhages. It has been used as a pot herb and in Spring cures. The seeds make an excellent tonic for birds.

SNOWDROP
(galanthus nivalis)

'Fair maid of February', one of the earliest and most delicate Spring flowers, this little white bell on its slender stalk is a common garden and wood-land flower. The bulbs are here used in a chilblain cure. They also occur in eye lotions.

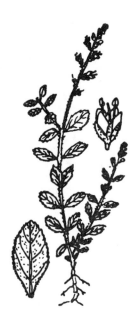

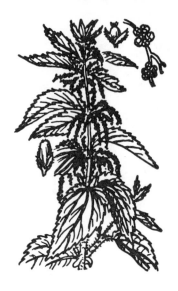

SPEEDWELL
(veronica officinalis)

This little creeping plant with its well known bright blue flowers grows everywhere, but prefers drier ground. It used to be used 'to improve the sight'. Its blue flowers like bright blue eyes invoked the doctrine of signatures but nowadays it is more generally used to treat catarrh and bronchial complaints. In cosmetics it is used in skin lotions.

STINGING NETTLES
(urtica dioica)

'Nettles are so well known that they need no description; they may be found by feeling in the darkest night'.
   Culpeper

Nevertheless I have included nettles in this herb list as many people do not realize what a useful plant it is. Campbell says:
'In Scotland, I have eaten nettles, I have slept in nettle sheets, and I have dined off a nettle table-cloth. The young and tender nettle is an excellent pot herb. The stalks of the old nettle are as good as flax for making a cloth'. Nettle pudding and nettle beer were also popular recipes and it has been used in dyes, cheesemaking and as a fodder crop.

Medically nettles make an excellent tonic and blood-purifier. The two nettle hair tonics given in this book are but a selection of the various hair rinses made with this plant.

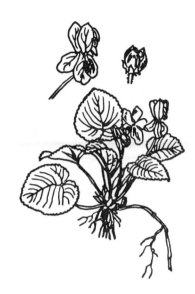

SWEET VIOLET
(viola odorata)

A violet by a mossy stone,
Half hidden from the eye.
  William Wordsworth

Violet 'the symbol of modesty' does indeed hide
itself from the casual observer. It grows in shady
moist places hanging its deep purple head towards
the shiny dark green leaves. It flowers in March
and has a very characteristic sweet perfume.
Although wild violets are still found all over the
British Isles it is becoming a popular garden plant
and can be purchased at many nurseries. It is
propagated from its runners. Violets were, and in
some places still are, widely used in cookery, both
for their perfume and colour which is imparted to
liquids. Syrup of violets had long been used as a
mild laxative for children and were used on
plasters as a 'wound' herb. One-time readers of
Little Grey Rabbit will remember her use of violet
plasters and violet smelling salts. In this book it is
used in pot pourris and face lotions.

THYME
(thymus vulgaris)

I know a bank whereon the wild thyme blows
Where oxslips and the nodding violet grows,
  A Midsummer Night's Dream

Thyme is a low growing, woody perennial plant
with small hard leaves and labiate mauve flowers.
But it is the scent that makes this such an
attractive plant. Anyone who has ever walked over
the moors on a warm sunny summer day, smelt
the enticing odour of wild thyme *(thymus
serpyllum)* and listened to the bees buzzing around
them will feel a deep affection for this small
aromatic plant.

Garden thyme has an even more intense perfume
and there are many interesting varieties, including
orange thyme, lemon thyme and caraway thyme.
Eleanour Sinclair Rohde mentions an old description of a garden near Dorking: 'There are 21 sorts
of thyme in the garden which may seem a second
Eden — where under heaven can be a sweeter
place?' Thyme grows well near lavender and also
likes a light, warm soil. In exposed situations it
will need protection from frost in the winter. This
herb does not like a polluted atmosphere and is
difficult to grow in town gardens.

Culpeper said that thyme 'is a noble strengthener
of the lungs' and it is still used in many cough
medicines. Thymol, which is extracted from
thyme, is a powerful antiseptic and thyme is sometimes added to creams and lotions for its antiseptic
qualities.

VALERIAN
(Valeriana officinalis)

This wayside flower grows to 3—4 feet in height
and is easily recognised in summer by its
compound head of pale pink flowers which have a
soft fluffy appearance. The leaves are 2—3 inches
long and arranged in pairs. Each leaf is formed by
pairs of leaflets. The dried rhizome is the part of
the plant used medically. This has a heavy,
sickening smell which has a very strange effect on **99**

cats who seem to get 'high' on it. It has the opposite effect on humans. It makes a very effective tranquillizer and a harmless but efficient sleeping draught. It was used by the old herbalists for treating epilepsy.

WHITE DEAD-NETTLE
(lamium album)

The dead-nettle owes its name to its resemblance to the stinging nettles. It is 'dead' because it has no sting. It is however no relation to the stinging nettle although it grows in similar places, on waste ground everywhere. It blooms from May to October and its white labial flowers grow in dense whorls at the axil of the leaves. Medically it is used in the treatment of catarrh and for female disorders. It is used in cosmetics for its softening qualities.

WITCH HAZEL
(hamamelis virginica)

This shrub grows ten to twelve feet in height. It produces several crooked branching trunks from one root. It is deciduous, but the clusters of yellow flowers do not appear until the leaves have been shed. Witch hazel is a native of North America and will not produce the edible nuts in this country, but it makes an ornamental garden plant as well as being useful medically and cosmetically.

Hamamelis is very astringent and will stop bleeding internally or externally. It is extensively used in the treatment of piles and as a household remedy for burns and inflammations. Cosmetically it is very important. An infusion can be prepared from the fresh leaves or a decoction from the dried bark and leaves.

WORMWOOD
(artemesia absinthium)

This is a bitter aromatic herb which contains the basic ingredient for 'absinthe', that alcoholic scourge of nineteenth-century France. It is a fairly common wayside plant and can be found growing on wasteground, especially by the sea. The flowering stem grows 2 to 2½ feet high and both it and its leaves are covered with fine soft hairs which give it a whitish colour. The ragged leaves are about 3 inches long. The little flowers appear in July until October and are greenish-yellow and pendulous. It is easily grown in a shady place in the garden. Wormwood has for centuries been used as a digestive and is very good for flatulence.

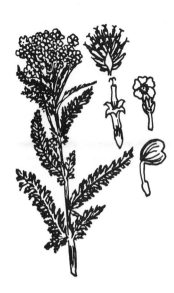

YARROW
(achillea millefolium)

Eldest of worts
Thou hast might for three
And against thirty
For venom availest
For flying vile thing
Mighty against loathed ones
That through the land rove.
  Harleian Ms. AD 585

Yarrow grows everywhere. In Dutch it is called appropriately 'thousand leaves'. Its feathery grey-green leaves are covered with a fine down and it produces flat compound heads of pale mauve or white daisylike flowers. It is an old witch's herb and it was said that the coupie who carried yarrow on their wedding day would have 7 happy years. There is a legend which says that its medical value was discovered by Achilles, a follower of the centaur Chiron. Nowadays it is used for feverish colds. It is used in hair lotions for dandruff and seborrhoea.

27 GLOSSARY OF OILS, FATS AND OTHER UNFAMILIAR SUBSTANCES

All these substances can be obtained from health food stores or drug stores, particularly those specialising in homeopathy.

Ambergris — a wax-like substance produced in the intestine of the sperm whale

Arnica — *Arnica montana*, a herb indigenous to the mountainous region of Central Europe. It is used in many folk remedies and is an important ingredient of various bruise oils and creams

Beeswax — yellow wax secreted by bees to build honeycombs

Benzoin tincture — tincture of the resin of the benzoin tree, *styrax benzoin*, grown in Thailand and parts of Indonesia

Bergamot oil — an essential oil made from the rind of the fruit of the bergamot, a small citrus tree

Castile soap — pure white unperfumed soap made from olive oil

Castor oil — as the *Concise Oxford Dictionary* says 'a nauseous vegetable oil used as a purgative' and in some face creams and tanning creams

Cocoa butter — a fatty substance obtained from cocoa beans

Fuller's earth — an absorbent purified clay

Glycerine — colourless sweet liquid obtained from animal and vegetable fatty substances by saponification

Gum tragacanth — also called gum dragon, the resin of a Near-Eastern shrub, *astralgus gummifer*

Lanolin — a purified fat extracted from sheep's wool

Peruvian balsam — extract from the fruit of the *myroxylon percirae*, a Central American tree, used in nose drops etc

Peruvian bark — bark of a South American tree, *cinchona succirubra*, cultivated in India and Java for its medical uses

Spermaceti — a hardening agent used in candle making and in many face creams. It is derived from the whale's head. Vegetarians will want to avoid creams made with this or any of the other animal-derived substances mentioned here

White wax — highly refined and purified beeswax

28 HERBAL SUPPLIERS

Fresh herb plants

Caprilands Herb Farm
Silver Street
Coventry, Connecticut 06238

Casa Yerba
Box 176
Tustin, California 92680

Gilbertie Florists of Westport
7 Sylvan Avenue
Westport, Connecticut 06883

Horticulture House
347 E. 55 Street
New York, New York 10022

Indiana Botanic Gardens
626 Seventeenth Street
Hammond, Indiana 46239

Nichols Garden Nursery
1190 North Pacific Highway
Albany, Oregon 97321

The Wide World of Herbs, Ltd.
11 St. Catherine Street East
Montreal, 129, Canada

Essential oils

Aphrodisia
28 Carmine Street
New York, New York 10014

Caswell-Massey Co., Ltd.
Catalogue-Order Department
320 West 13th Street
New York, New York 10014

Lanolin, oils, waxes, cocoa butter, fuller's earth,
kaolin powder, alum, borax, distilled water, etc.

Most drugstores or ordered from Caswell-Massey

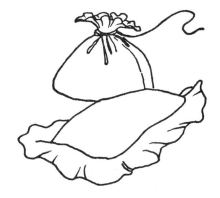

29 BIBLIOGRAPHY

OTHER BOOKS ON HERBS AND BEAUTY

Buchman, Dian Dincin. *The Complete Herbal Guide to Natural Health and Beauty*. New York, New York: Doubleday, 1973.

Castleton, Virginia. *Secrets of Natural Beauty*. New Canaan, Connecticut: Keats Publishing, Inc., 1977.

Clark, Linda, and others. *Your Natural Beauty Sampler*. New Canaan, Connecticut: Keats Publishing, Inc., 1977.

Harris, Ben Charles. *The Compleat Herbal*. New York, New York: Larchmont Books, 1972. *Eat the Weeds*. New Canaan, Connecticut: Keats Publishing, Inc., 1973.

Loewenfeld, Claire and Back, Philippa. *The Complete Books of Herbs and Spices*. New York, New York: G.P. Putnam's Sons, 1974.

Nature's Big Beautiful Bountiful Feel-Good Book. Ed. by *Health Quarterly*. New Canaan, Connecticut: Keats Publishing, Inc., 1977.

Rose, Jeanne, *Herbs & Things*. New York, New York: Grosset & Dunlap, 1973.

The *Living with Herbs* series published by Keats Publishing, Inc., New Canaan, Connecticut

Volume 1 Herbs, Health and Astrology by Leon Petulengro

Volume 2 Choosing, Planting and Cultivating Herbs by Philippa Back

Volume 3 Growing Herbs as Aromatics by Roy Genders

Volume 4 Making Things with Herbs by Elizabeth Walker

Volume 5 Herbs for Making Natural Soaps and Cosmetics by Alyson Huxley

Volume 6 Herbs in a Healthy House by Philippa Back

INDEX

Almond oil, in cord cream, 17
almond oil cream, 17
in honey cream, 17
in orange blossom cream, 18
eye make-up remover, 23
in cleansing creams, 24
in anti-wrinkle cream, 33
for wrinkles, 33
for eye lashes, 39
in face mask, 42
bath, 44
hair massage, 58
for hands, 51, 62
for finger nails, 63
Aloes, bitter, to prevent nail-biting, 63
Ambergris, in eau de Cologne, 72
in lavender water, 72
Angelica, in mouthwash, 35
Anise, in mouthwash, 35
Arnica, tincture in hair lotion, 48
hair rinse, 50
Artichoke, for slimming, 75
in slimming tea, 75
Aubergine, for freckles, 37
Avocado, face mask, 42

Balm, in complexion lotion, 21
in 17th-century herbal bath, 45
Barley meal, in face mask, 42
Beech, inner bark for pimples, 28
Beer, hair rinse, 51
Beetroot, for wrinkles, 33
face mask, 42
Benzoin tincture, in winter hand lotion, 63
Bergamot oil, in sun oil, 31
in eau de Cologne, 72
in lavender water, 72
Betony, spots and pimples, 27
Bilberry, cosmetic uses, 13

Birch, for spots and pimples, 27
in hair lotion, 49
in hair rinses, 50
in herbal shampoo, 59
for slimming, 75
Blackberry, in complexion lotion, 22
foot deodorant, 65
Bladderwrack, for slimming, 74
in slimming bath, 75
in slimming tea, 75
Borage, for spots and pimples, 27, 28
Burdock, for spots and pimples, 27
in depurative tea, 28
hair rinse, 50
Buttermilk, cleanser, 23
for sunburn, 31
for freckles, 37
compress, 42
body packs, 43

Cabbage, complexion lotion, 21
sauerkraut juice hair rinse, 51
sauerkraut juice for slimming, 75
Camomile, cosmetic uses, 14
complexion lotion, 21
for sunburn, 31
for eyes, 39
in eyebrow mixture, 40
bath, 44
hair lotion, 48
hair rinse, 50
hair colourant, 52
in blond hair rinse, 54
shampoo for blond hair, 55
to keep hands soft, 61
in foot bath, 66
for slimming, 74
in slimming tea, 75

Caraway, in pot pourri, 72
Carrot, juice in lotions, 27
    for spots and pimples, 26
    compresses, 27
    for tanning, 30
Castile soap, in cleansing cream, 24
    in shampoo for blond hair, 55
    in herbal shampoo, 59
Castor oil, in cream, 17
    in eyelash pomade, 40
    in hair lotion, 48
Cherry, stalks in slimming tea, 75
Cherry laurel, in stimulating tonic, 20
Chickweed, complexion lotion, 22
    for spots and pimples, 27
    for slimming, 74
Chillies, for hair, 15
    hair lotion, 48
    hair rinse, 51
Cider vinegar, for dandruff, 59
Cinnamon, in mouthwash, 35
    in pot pourri, 71
Citrus medica, in eau de Cologne, 72
Cleavers, in hair rinse, 51
    for slimming, 74
Cloves, in mouthwash, 35
    in pomander, 71
    in pot pourri, 72
Clover, red, lip salve, 36
Clover, white, in complexion lotion, 22
    in bark and blossom drink, 28
Cocoa butter, eye wrinkle cream, 40
Coconut butter, cleansing cream, 24
Coconut oil, for tanning, 30
    in sun oil, 31
    in anti-wrinkle cream, 33
Coltsfoot, cosmetic uses, 14
    for spots and pimples, 26
    hair rinse, 50
Cornflour, in face mask, 42
Cornflower, eye compress, 39
    in eyebrow mixture, 40
Cowslip, for wrinkles, 33
Cream, face mask with fruit, 42
    face mask with beetroot or potato, 42
    for chilblains, 62
Cucumber, cosmetic uses, 14
    in orange and lemon tonic, 19
    in skin tonic, 19

    in milk cleanser, 23
    skin cleanser, 23
    for freckles, 37
    and egg mask, 42
Daisy, complexion lotion, 22
    for chilblains, 66
Dandelion, leaves for spots and pimples, 27
    juice for pimples, 27, 28
    for slimming, 75
    in slimming bath, 75
    in slimming tea, 75

Egg, in honey cream, 17
    in anti-freckle cream, 38
    yolk and lemon mask, 41
    face mask, 42
    astringent mask, 42
    and yeast face pack, 42
    and fruit mask, 42
    and lemon body pack, 43
    shampoo, 58
    for chilblains, 62
Elder, flowers in cucumber tonic, 19
    flowers in complexion lotions, 22
    leaves for spots and pimples, 27
    inner bark in bark and blossom drink, 28
    flowers for sunburn, 31
    for freckles, 22
    berries for hair colourant, 53
    flower hand lotion, 62, 63
Eucalyptus, hand rinse, 61

Fennel, seeds for eye bath, 39
    for slimming, 74
    in slimming tea, 75
Fig, chilblain ointment, 67
Fuller's earth, face mask, 41
Fumitory, in eyebrow mixture, 40

Garlic, for wrinkles, 33
    hair lotion, 48
    tips for hair, 58
Gelatine, and orange drink for fingernails, 63
Glycerine, for hands, 61
    hand jelly, 62
    in lemon hand lotion, 62
    in elderflower hand lotion, 63
    for finger nails, 63

Grapefruit, in complexion lotion, 21
Greater celandine, for corns, 65
Ground almonds, cleanser, 23
    face mask, 42
Groundsel, hand rinse, 61
Gum tragacanth, in hand jelly, 62

Hawthorn, in complexion lotion, 22
    leaves for spots and pimples, 28
Hazel, cosmetic uses, 13
    hand rinse, 61
    for chilblains, 62
Henna, hair colourant, 53
Honey, cream, 17
    and egg white face mask, 42
Honeysuckle, bath, 44
Horse chestnut, for chilblains, 65
Horseradish, for blotches and freckles, 37
Horsetail, for hair, 15
    for eyes, 39
    healing bath, 44
    hair rinse, 50
    for fingernails, 63
    in slimming bath, 75

Iris, orris powder, 70
    in pot pourri, 71
    in pomander, 71

Jasmine, hair rinse, 51

Lady's bedstraw, foot bath, 65
Lanolin, nourishing face cream, 18
    anti-wrinkle cream, 33
    hand cream, 62
Lavender, in bark and blossom drink, 28
    sun oil, 31
    mouthwash, 34
    bath, 44
    in mixed herbal bath, 44
    in 17th-century herbal bath, 45
    in herbal bath oil, 46
    bath extract, 46
    hair lotion, 48
    hair rinse, 51
    for hands, 61
    hand lotion, 62
    perfume, 70
    pot pourri, 72

    water, 72
    vinaigre de lavande, 73
Lemon, cosmetic uses, 13
    in skin tonic, 19
    in complexion lotion, 21
    to strengthen gums, 34
    for freckles, 37
    in anti-freckle cream, 38
    and egg yolk face mask, 41, 42
    and eggwhite in face mask, 42
    and orange body pack, 43
    and milk body pack, 43
    and egg in body pack, 43
    hair colourants, 52
    shampoo, 55
    hair rinse, 59
    hand lotion, 61, 62
    for fingernails, 63
    in eau de Cologne, 72
Lemon balm, see Balm
Lemon verbena, complexion lotion, 21
    to clean teeth, 32
Lime, for freckles, 37
    in eye compress, 39
    hair rinse, 50
Lovage, complexion lotion, 21
    for spots and pimples, 27
    deodorant bath, 44
Lupin, bath, 44

Maidenhair fern, hair rinse, 51
Maize, hair in slimming tea, 75
Marigold, cosmetic uses, 14
    complexion lotion, 22
    in bark and blossom drink, 28
    hair colourant, 52
Marjoram, mixed herbal bath, 44
    in 17th-century bath, 45
    in herbal bath oil, 46
    in foot bath, 66
Marsh-mallow, cosmetic uses, 14
    in complexion lotion, 21
Meadowsweet, in depurative tea, 28
Milk, cleanser, 23
    and cucumber cleanser, 23
    and spinach face mask, 42
    body pack, 43
    compress, 42
Mistletoe, for pimples, 27

Mugwort, for pimples, 28

Nettle, *see* Stinging nettle

Oak, leaf deodorant bath, 44
    hand rinse, 61
    foot deodorant, 65
Oatmeal, cleanser, 23
    in face mask, 42
    body pack, 43
    bath, 46
    for hands, 61
Olive oil, for tanning, 30
    in sun oil, 31
    in lavender sun oil, 31
    and vinegar sun oil, 30
    in anti-freckle cream, 38
    for eye lashes, 39
    and egg yolk face mask, 42
    hair massage, 58
    for hands, 61
    for finger nails, 63
Onion, for hair, 58
    for corns, 65, 66
Orange, and lemon tonic, 19
    in complexion lotion, 21
    and egg yolk face mask, 42
    and lemon body pack, 43
    and glycerine for finger nails, 63
    for pomanders, 71
    oil in eau de Cologne, 72
Orange blossom, face cream, 18
    in stimulating tonic, 20
    skin tonic, 20
    complexion lotion, 21
    in bath extract, 46
Orris powder, *see* Iris

Parsley, for freckles, 37
Peach, face mask, 42
Peanut oil, and castor oil cream, 17
Pennyroyal, in 17th-century herbal bath, 45
Pennywort, for spots and pimples, 27
Peppermint, bath, 44
    in 17th-century herbal bath, 45
    in foot bath, 66
    in pot pourri, 72
Peruvian balsam, in hair lotion, 48
    in winter hand lotion, 63

Peruvian bark, in hair lotions, 48
    in hair rinse, 50
Pine, bath extract, 45
Plantain, cosmetic uses, 13
    for spots and pimples, 27
Potato, for wrinkles, 33
    face mask, 42
    cream hand lotion, 62
Primrose, for freckles, 37
    for wrinkles, 33
Privet, hair colourant, 53
Pumpkin, for freckles, 38

Quince, emollient for sunburn, 31
    hair colourant, 52

Rainwater, cleanser, 23
Raspberry, leaves for pimples, 28
Rhubarb, in blond hair rinse, 54
Rose, water and witch hazel tonic, 19
    in complexion lotion, 22
    cleanser, 23
    oil in lip salve, 36
    bath, 44
    in hair rinse, 51
    in hand jelly, 62
    perfume, 69
    in pot pourri, 71
    in slimming tea, 75
Rose geranium, in pot pourri, 71
Rosemary, for hair, 15, 39
    skin tonic, 20
    in complexion lotion, 22
    for wrinkles, 33
    toothpowder, 34
    mouthwash, 34
    for freckles, 37
    in anti-freckle cream, 38
    in eye wrinkle cream, 40
    bath, 44
    in mixed herbal bath, 44
    hair rinse, 50
    in hair lotions, hair colourant, 53
    shampoo, 55, 59
    in foot bath, 65, 66
    perfume, 69, 71
    for slimming, 75
Rum, hair tonic, 48
    grey hair lotion, 54

St John's wort, cosmetic uses, 14
    in moisturising compress, 42
    in camomile hair lotion, 48
Sage, toothpowder, 34
    in chapped lip ointment, 36
    in depurative tea, 29
    in mixed herbal bath, 44
    cream for cold sores, 36
    in eyebrow mixture, 40
    in grey hair rinse, 54
    hair colourant, 53
    shampoo, 55, 59
    for slimming, 75
Salt, to clean teeth, 34
    to rinse hair, 59
    in pot pourri, 72
    for slimming, 74
Sauerkraut, *see* Cabbage
Savory, for spots and pimples, 27
Scarlet pimpernel, for freckles, 37
Self heal, for spots, pimples and cold sores, 27
Sesame oil, in nourishing face cream, 18
    for tanning, 30
    in sun oil, 31
Shepherd's purse, for spots and pimples, 27
Snowdrop, in chilblain ointment, 67
Speedwell, complexion lotion, 21
    for spots and pimples, 27
Spermaceti, in cold cream, 17
    in nourishing face cream, 18
    in anti-wrinkle cream, 33
    in chapped lip ointment, 36
    in anti-freckle cream, 38
Spinach, for spots and pimples, 27
    face mask, 42
Stinging nettle, for hair, 15, 48
    in depurative tea, 28
    in hair lotions, 48
    in herbal shampoo, 59
Strawberry, face mask, 42
    in mouthwash, 34
Sunflower oil, to replace almond oil, 12
Sweet violet, cleansing milk, 24
    lip salve, 36
    hair rinse, 51

Tea, hair colourant, 52
    hair rinse, 54
Tobacco, hair colourant, 53

Tomato, for freckles, 37
Thyme, in complexion lotion, 22
    in mouthwash, 35
    in mixed herbal bath, 44
    in 17th-century herbal bath, 45
    in herbal bath oil, 46
    in herbal shampoo, 59
    in foot bath, 66
    in pot-pourri, 72
    for slimming, 75

Valerian, bath, 44
Vaseline, with marigolds, 14
    cleansing cream, 24
    in eyelash pomade, 40
    in hand cream, 62
Verbena, *see* Lemon verbena
Vinegar, to rinse hair, 59
Violet, *see* Sweet violet

Walnut, juice in eyelash pomade, 40
    in hair colourant, 54
Watercress, for spots and pimples, 27, 28
Wheatgerm oil, for eye wrinkles, 40
White dead-nettle, in depurative tea, 28
    for sunburn, 31
    in eyebrow mixture, 40
White wine, for sunburn, 31
    mouthwash, 20
    in nettle lotion, 48
Witch hazel, and rosewater tonic, 19
    for shiny nose, 35
    eye compress, 39
Wormwood, in 17th-century herbal bath, 45

Yarrow, for hair, 15, 39
    in complexion lotion, 21
    in hair rinse, 50
    in herbal shampoo, 59
Yeast, and egg face mask, 42
Yoghurt, compress, 42
    body pack, 43

NOTES AND RECIPES

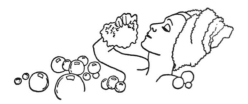

Use these last pages for your personal natural-beauty history. When you try the recipes in this book, keep a record of how they worked for you. Experiment with ingredient changes and note down how that goes. Read other books on natural beauty and copy recipes that interest you into this section.

Remember, you are unique and your own beauty book should be, too!

NOTES AND RECIPES

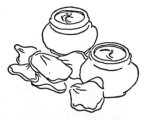

NOTES AND RECIPES

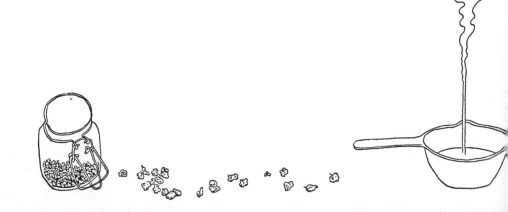

NOTES AND RECIPES

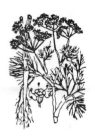

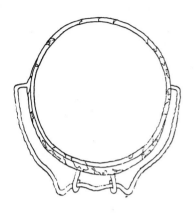

NOTES AND RECIPES

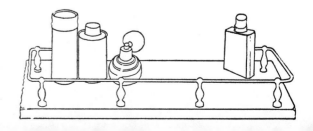

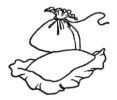

NOTES AND RECIPES

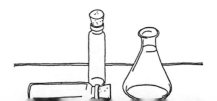

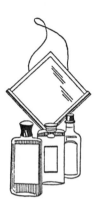

NOTES AND RECIPES

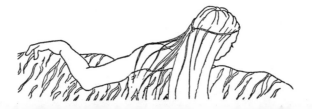

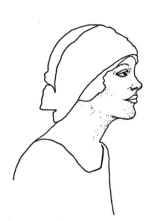